Don't Mention Dementia

Jack Bennington

chipmunkapublishing
the mental health publisher

All rights reserved, no part of this publication may be reproduced by any means, electronic, mechanical photocopying, documentary, film or in any other format without prior written permission of the publisher.

Published by

Chipmunkapublishing

PO Box 6872

Brentwood

Essex CM13 1ZT

United Kingdom

http://www.chipmunkapublishing.com

Copyright © Jack Bennington 2012

Edited by Aleks Lech

ISBN   978-1-84991-796-4

Chipmunkapublishing gratefully acknowledge the support of Arts Council England.

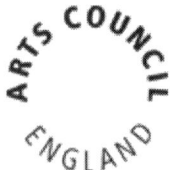

Jack Bennington

For Jackie & Larry

Don't Mention Dementia

Jack Bennington

Thanks to:

V.M for continued inspiration and confidence,

P.W for keeping my spirits up,

H.M.P for being supportive,

E.P for the supervision and green tea,

and to all my residents, past and present,

without whom this book could not have been.

Don't Mention Dementia

Author Biography

Jack Bennington was born in the Midlands in 1977. He gained a degree in media, but after developing an interest in psychology, later trained as a mental health nurse. Upon qualifying he took up a position working with individuals with dementia.

Jack continues to develop his interest and knowledge of mental health issues, exploring links between healthy living, psychology, and the mind. He still tries to work closely with his local university in developing educational and visual training tools for future mental health students.

By the same author:

Mental Health: A Student Nurse Account

Don't Mention Dementia

The following characters, identities and location names have been changed to protect anonymity and confidentiality. In no way is this book intended to make fun of mental health care or people with a mental health illness. This book is not a work of fiction. The home in question is a real working home; all the events and situations described in the book are fact, and serve to highlight the working environment in a typical private nursing home, and the experiences and challenges that I have faced working as a newly qualified mental health nurse.

You will learn about mental health and dementia care, which will help inform and educate. It has been necessary to incorporate some theory alongside some situations experienced to support my actions.

Working within dementia care can be tough, being both challenging but also highly rewarding. The following encapsulates a year working within the home, told over a typical twelve hour shift. It begins with my own trepidation as I face my first day, and includes views and opinions developed with the benefit of hindsight. This provides added depth to my account and shows you that there is hope for the future of dementia care.

This book will show you dementia, up close and personal, and the real people behind the illness. It will show that we continually need to be looking at the person as a whole and remove the stigma attached to dementia. Patients with dementia are often people who have lived long and fulfilling lives with stories, experiences and wisdom that we can still learn from if we choose to listen correctly.

I offer you this book as an insight into the complexities involved with working closely with a wide range of people from varying backgrounds and life experience, who have at times forgotten who they are. It is up to us to remind them.

Let us start getting back to person centred care and chip away at the stigma and labelling that appears to manifest itself in mental health. As my lecturer once told me, *'we can only do what we can, one bit at a time, and make a difference one small step each day.'*

I hope you enjoy the following; I certainly had an adventure living and experiencing it.

The name Jack Bennington is a pseudonym.

Jack Bennington
London, 2011

Prologue

Chapter 1	8 – 9 a.m.
Chapter 2	9 – 10 a.m.
Chapter 3	10 – 11 a.m.
Chapter 4	11 – 12 p.m.
Chapter 5	12 – 1 p.m.
Chapter 6	1 – 2 p.m.
Chapter 7	2 – 3 p.m.
Chapter 8	3 – 4 p.m.
Chapter 9	4 – 5 p.m.
Chapter 10	5 – 6 p.m.
Chapter 11	6 – 7 p.m.
Chapter 12	7 – 8 p.m.

Epilogue

Don't Mention Dementia

"Dementia is a syndrome due to disease of the brain, usually of a chronic or progressive nature, in which there is disturbance of multiple higher cortical functions, including memory, thinking, orientation, comprehension, calculation, learning capacity, language, and judgement."

World Health Organisation, (1993)

'The more you read and learn,

the less your adversary will know.'

Sun Tzu

Prologue

A person's life begins when they are born. They grow up, and have a wealth of life experiences; they meet people along the way. Some get married, some have children. But it is their life. They choose to live it how they want. Whatever happens, they retain that life experience, and they are an individual on this planet, with their own unique experience and outlook on the world.

What is your definition of Mental Health? What images does it conjure up in your head? Place those images firmly in the forefront of your mind. Imagine them projected onto a huge cinema screen, vivid and colourful. Take a few minutes to watch those images scroll past. Remember them clearly.

I am a mental health nurse. For some of you, you may have an idea of what this entails; for everyone else, you will be none the wiser. After the events of this book, you will have a further appreciation and understanding of the challenges and work that goes into the role, and discover what a mental health nurse does, day in, day out. Welcome to the next twelve hours of my life.

I remember thinking for years, like most other people, that nursing was really women's work, and nurses must spend all their time walking around hospital beds, emptying bed pans, and generally just being nice. This was a terribly misogynistic outlook, and one I now realise was completely inaccurate.

I never thought that I would ever become a nurse, let alone a mental health nurse. I guess in the past I had held a very blinkered view of mental illness as being 'scary' and 'dangerous'. I would often glance at a newspaper and see the headlines glaring back at me,

'Schizophrenic murdered entire family.' 'Manic Depressive burgled elderly lady's home.' 'Local woman jumps off multi storey car park.' I, like others, developed a very negative impression of mental health.

What had opened my eyes to mental health had all started during a bleak midwinter day at an open day at my local university. I had decided to attend a two day taster session, during which I experienced some sample lectures and a brief introduction to what mental health nursing was all about, giving me an insight into what would be required of me if I were to embark on this career path. I went away from this feeling enthusiastic and inspired. It had shown me how varied a career in mental health could be, and as I bid goodbye to fellow attendees I wondered if I would ever see them or the university again, but things were about to change for me.

Fast forward three years later....

It almost didn't seem real. As I glanced at my letter from the Nursing and Midwifery Council (NMC), it slowly sank in. I had done it. I had gone through three years of RMN (Registered Mental Nurse) training. At times it had been an uphill struggle, and on numerous occasions I had thought of quitting the course when it had seemed like I wasn't getting anywhere, but I persevered.

I kept pressing on with what I hoped would eventually be worth all the late nights, all the stress over the examinations, all the assignments, and continual bickering and disagreements during group work and presentations. I figured I really had to take charge of my life. I felt that I had to make sure I had a particular set of skills that would help me make a difference in my life, and ultimately, other people's lives. The letter that I had opened this morning had confirmed that I had passed, with merit no less. It was official now, there was no going back, this was three years of my life in my hands. I could now place the letters RMN after my name.

It wasn't that long ago that I was on my final placement area wondering when it would end, counting down the days until the end of the placement. Having worked on a dementia ward in a hospital setting, this had really put me off working for my local trust. It appeared that the patients didn't always get the best of what they should be getting. I put all that behind me and made the decision not to apply for the jobs that had been offered. They were only six month contracts anyway, due to start in April. It was now January, snow and ice was on the ground and my wallet was empty. I wasn't waiting around for a job until April. A six month contract wasn't enough time to get involved in a job before having to worry about where the next pay cheque was going to come from. No, I'd made the right decision. I struck out on my own.

Dementia will continue to be a growing area of Mental Health. As we are all living longer and healthier lives, this has a massive impact on our older population. Dementia is set to continue to be a huge growth area that will have immense cost implications for the Government.

I had attended the interview only a few days ago, and, as horrible as interviews are, this was perhaps the strangest I had ever experienced. Looking back, there seemed an air of desperation in the meeting, although the home itself was beautifully appointed. There hadn't been any taxing questions asked at all. I mainly just talked about myself and showed the manager what additional qualifications I had completed during my nurse training. After that it was 'When can you start?' and 'How many shifts do you want?' It made me feel good to be wanted all of a sudden. The manager had bluntly stated that I could 'use them for the experience, then just move on' if I so wished.

After years of dead end jobs, here I was, a professional. I had actually been offered three jobs in quick succession, this one, a second one in another home but much further away and a third working with young adults. With the third I would have been the only nurse in charge of medication with overall general responsibility for the running of the six bed unit. I wasn't prepared for that much responsibility so soon in my career so I turned it down.

I had opted for the private nursing home closest to home. At the end of the day I needed work, and I needed it quickly. It was time to start the new adventure and leave the horrible memories of working within the hospital setting behind me. I could still hear the faint patronising voice of Nurse Linda, who always used to call me 'luvee' and took perverse delight in trying to break my spirit with menial tasks which she supervised, waiting for me to fail or do it wrong, feeling under constant pressure, like a dog on a leash for the duration of the shift. Thinking back to those days always brought a shudder.

My lecturers were right. They had told me I would never be out of a job working in mental health, and the prophecy appeared to have come true. I looked up at my year planner in front of me and carefully marked with a thick black marker January 5th, the day on which I would start my new 'career for life'. I had no idea what to expect, but I was sure it would be an adventure, whatever happened.

8–9 a.m.

It had felt like I was sitting on a plane, ready for take-off, the engines roaring, my seat belt securely fastened, and my hands gripping tightly onto my chair, a few beads of sweat glistening on my hands and face, waiting for the pilot to take my life into his hands. One of those days where I felt like just crawling back into bed and forgetting everything.

Today marked the first day of my new job as a mental health nurse at a private nursing home. Elderly care was not my first choice for a job, it was working on a dementia unit, and I was prepared for the worst. Most residents were in their eighties and nineties, and most had come from a psychiatric hospital or home. The average length of time a resident stayed was roughly eighteen months. This was end stage dementia. Our goal here was to make the residents as comfortable as possible and provide them with the best quality of life for their final years.

During my interview I'd received a tour of the facility. At the time it had seemed a 'flagship home'; newly built with state of the art modern conveniences including fifty inch LCD televisions in the lounge areas, and individual flat screens and en-suite facilities in each of the residents' rooms. All the carpets looked new, and smelled nice. I had toured around a few other nursing homes in my time and there were some truly awful looking ones, which all seemed to smell like the mustiness found in charity shops, underpinned with an ever present lingering odour of stale urine.

I had no uniform or papers with me except for the initial letter of acceptance confirming my appointment with the company. It was finally time to replace my 'student nurse' badge which was still lying on my bedside table.

I was due to start at eight every morning, but this first morning, I was up bright and early. I felt like I'd barely been able to sleep the night before. I had a few night terrors, dreaming of old lunatic asylums and patients trying to kill me with axes and other unsavoury sharp implements.

I had no idea if I was going to get a uniform immediately today, so I played it safe and opted for a dark blue polo shirt and the usual black Nike trainers. May as well be comfortable I thought, as I had no idea as to what would be expected of me today. I hoped I wouldn't be put in charge so early on. I needed to complete a drugs assessment and understand the running of the unit before I could be in charge anyway, so I imagined (and hoped) the first few weeks would be available to just settle in, meet the residents and get used to everything.

I made myself a coffee and walked out of the kitchen, staring longingly at a canvas picture of New York City above my sofa. I aimed to go back soon. I tried to remind myself that this is why I had chosen to take the job, amongst other things; everyone needed a source of income, and without one I sure as hell wouldn't be able to visit New York again.

There were still remnants of Christmas decorations around the house. Piles of cards lay strewn on the glass coffee table in the lounge, ready to be locked away in the attic. Odd bits of green glittery tinsel could still be spotted on the carpet.

Once I had gulped down my coffee, I re-check my bag and go upstairs for one final bathroom check. I look at myself in the mirror and wonder if I had done the right thing. You don't get anywhere in this life without a bit of risk and a sense of adventure, so I thought what the hell, what's the worst that could happen? With this in mind, I set off for my first shift.

Clearing ice from the car in the bitter cold really didn't do my nerves much good. Swearing as my fingers began to lose sensitivity I attempted to remain cheerful.

I loaded a Foo Fighters album into the car stereo. This is my soundtrack to the morning. The home is only a twenty minute drive, but I allowed myself a good thirty five minutes this morning.

The drive is cold and miserable; not many people about, just the odd person walking a dog. I'm taking it nice and slow. The car is heating up and Dave Grohl's dulcet tones over the speakers provided a sense of calm.

The home is tucked away down a huge lane off the beaten track from the main road, ironically not far away from where I had done a lot of my training in a psychiatric hospital, the one which had been the setting for my previous night terrors.

As I turned right at the mini roundabout, I glanced over to my left and could just see one of the corners of the hospital, which still sent shivers down my spine, thinking of Nurse Linda shouting out her orders to me as a lowly student nurse and making my life a living hell for the entirety of each shift.

I drove slowly down the long lane. It seemed to take forever. I eventually parked up in the car park, and sat for a few minutes. The home was only two years old, and it was split onto two levels. Each level had two units per floor, housing a total capacity of eighty residents. There were only two dementia units; the other units were focused on palliative care, end of life care for sufferers of varying forms of cancer, or elderly residents who had mobility problems and simply couldn't afford to live on their own any more without constant help and support.

The average price per week of this home was around eight to nine hundred pounds. At full capacity you were looking at over three million pounds a year turnover. Rumour had it that it was generally only the last few beds that really made the profit, which is why the home were always keen to quickly have each bed filled as soon as they could and maintain a 97.5% occupancy rate. Beds could be filled within a matter of hours at times. A resident could pass away at ten in the morning, and there could be a brand new resident, having his pants and socks put into his top drawer by twelve. There was a big waiting list for the home, and demand was only ever going to increase.

Most of the residents would be funded through various councils and funding bodies, unless they happened to have over twenty three thousand, two hundred and fifty pounds in savings or total assets. If their assets were higher than this, then they would be classed as self funding until the main bulk of their savings had been used up. This would not take that long given the prices of the home. This was a pretty standard figure across the whole country. Care costs. A lot.

I step out of my car, still feeling the bitter January morning, and walk towards the imposing building. There was a very large red button next to a keypad. I push the large big red button and step inside where there is a small but empty reception desk. Everything is bathed in a deep amber hue. It reminded me of a very posh hotel reception.

Before I had time to glance anywhere else, the home manager came walking up to me. She was actually the acting manager. I had no idea where the real manager was. The acting manager seemed nice enough; she had told me at the interview that she herself had only been qualified two years as a general nurse. She was of medium build with short blonde hair, cut fashionably, and her name was Jennifer. I would guess that she was in her early forties, and she had a distinct air of authority. She was carrying a small package under her arm.

'Jack!' she smiled. 'Here's your uniform, I hope it fits, I just had to guess what size you were. You are upstairs on Franklyn unit, the code is 1713; I'll come and see you later.'

She walked off through another corridor, in quite a hurry. I could remember vaguely being shown around upstairs, so I slowly walked up the pristine shiny wood panelled stairs, and around the corner. Everything was quite clearly labelled, but I couldn't get over how quiet everything all seemed. I walk through another set of double doors and a small carpeted area, until I get to the doors to Franklyn unit. I push the buttons on the keypad in front of me and, taking a deep breath, open the door.

The corridor was huge, wall to wall carpets in deep blue, and an eclectic mix of posters adorned the walls, from the Beatles to Elvis, alongside a large map of the United Kingdom. The corridor seemed to stretch on forever with no alternative exit in sight. I keep walking, passing the doors to the residents rooms two at a time on either side of the corridor. Most of the residents seemed to be in bed. Music is emanating from one of the residents' rooms. The tune was spilling out into the corridor, and creating a theme tune to my long walk. Johnny Cash's 'Solitary Man'.

I eventually pass the nurse's station. These always looked the same. A small cubby hole stacked with paper and a small office chair and computer. I walked past the station and towards the large lounge area. I could see a large gathering of people sat at the table in the far corner. There were four women all dressed in light blue uniforms and an older male dressed in dark blue. I walked up towards the table and introduced myself.

'Hi'

The older male turned to me first.

'Hiya mate, Jack isn't it? First day today is it?'

'Yeah, sure is' I say.

Grasping my hand in his, he pumped it firmly up and down in a surprisingly strong handshake.

'I'm Paul, pleased to meet you mate'. Paul must have been in his mid fifties. He had a dark brown beard with grey flecks, and small tinted spectacles on. His hair extended down to just above his shoulders. I liked him on sight.

Paul was from the 'old school' days of nursing; he had learnt his trade in the hospitals of the eighties. He had come to this home to keep his nursing registration going, and semi-retire. He worked a few days a week, and spent the rest of his time tending his garden and relaxing. I would come to realise that his experience in mental health and his wealth of knowledge would be a considerable asset to this home, and to a newbie like me.

Paul would eventually become my greatest confidante, and a true friend. We would come to work on some of the hardest shifts the home could throw at us, but we would get through it, with strength, determination, and good solid teamwork. Paul would be the workmate that you used to relish going to work to see, someone you would have a laugh with, but also someone to count on when you needed them most.

Paul extended his hand to the other ladies and introduced them all to me.

'This is Sharon, Jenny, Emma, and Katie.' They all greeted me.

Most were in their mid to late forties at my estimation. In my experience carers seemed to fall into two categories; they were either young, straight from college, or middle aged in their forties or fifties, usually working just to have a bit of pocket money for themselves. Of the older carers, the majority seemed pretty financially secure. Mortgages paid off, kids at university, or in work themselves, husbands either retired or in upper middle management roles. The younger carers would often discover that the care industry is not an easy line of work, and certainly not a job to pursue just for the money. It was a physically and mentally demanding job and life experience would be a useful tool.

I sat down at the table with them; each one of them had a steaming hot cup of very strong coffee which looked like mud in a mug to me. There was a sense of calm before the storm as we all sat there at the table.

I glanced around the lounge. I paid particular attention to the fifty inch LCD TV that was in the middle of it. The lounge had a mish-mash of chairs and tables, but they looked much comfier than the ones I'd seen in my earlier stint in the hospital. There were at least a dozen chairs lined up in the middle, in a rough semi circle. The rest of the chairs were lined up against the windows.

There were a few residents milling about in the lounge area. A very small and frail old lady with white hair sat in one of the chairs. She was moving her hand towards her mouth and making eating gestures, as though she was eating food only she could see. Her feet were tapping on the floor in a rhythmical pattern. She was very colour co-ordinated, dressed in a purple polka dot dress and matching purple cardigan, with bright stripy pink fluffy socks. She seemed very settled, eating her imaginary food, her eyes closed, tapping away to herself.

There was a younger looking gentleman sat in a chair nearer to our table. He had short black hair, greying at the sides, his eyes were also shut, but he seemed to be whistling to himself and tapping his feet. He kept making strange bird like sounds and staring up at the sky. Suddenly he made a very loud rasping noise like he was trying to clear his throat. I then realised he was actually gathering up large amounts of phlegm from the back of his throat. One of the carers shouted out.

'Andrew, stop it!'

Andrew either didn't hear this request or couldn't understand it. He continued with his throaty sounds and hawked out the phlegm across the lounge area, onto the floor.

The carer nearest me glanced in my direction.

'Don't worry, he does that a lot, just be careful!'

'Okay' I reply and try to break out a small smile. I had seen worse after all. Far worse.

Directly behind me was a large whiteboard. This appeared to be detailing who was on shift today; my name was there along with Paul's under the 'in charge' sub heading, and in brackets 'induction'. The rest of the carers' names were underneath. Beside each person's name was the shift pattern they were doing; we were all doing eight till eight today. The rest of the board was filled with the menu for lunch. Just below the whiteboard was a large silver coloured table, and at the far end, a sink. The lounge was very spacious; probably double the size of what you would get at a hospital. All around the far side of the room were large windows looking out onto the garden below.

I guessed from experience that this is where the handovers would be taking place, the daily debrief from the night staff, giving us a quick run-down of the previous nights shift, and any concerns that may need raising.

'Hey mate do you fancy a drink? We are just going to do handover in a few minutes, we've got plenty of time' Paul said.

'Sure, a coffee white no sugar would be great thanks' I replied. I didn't want to confuse everyone by getting out my supply of herbal teas. It was going to be far too complicated for such an early hour.

Paul stood up and walked off through the corridor past the nurse's station and turned right.

The carers and I make some small talk about how cold this January really is and how dark it is. They all seemed really friendly. Within a few minutes Paul had returned carrying two large mugs of coffee. He was whistling and singing to himself as he walked down the corridor.

'Baadda badda dum,' Paul chirped.

After more small talk with Paul and the rest of the carers it was time for handover. A lady was coming down the corridor past the nurse's station jangling a massive bunch of keys and holding a clipboard. I must say it was so good not to have to be cramped into a tiny little office doing handover as a student nurse and feeling awkward.

I still felt a little trepidation with the handover process. I was keeping an open mind today. The lady coming towards us was solidly built but had a friendly face and smile, with jet black hair styled in a neat bob. She sat down at the head of the table and let out a large sigh. She was visibly tired. No matter where I had worked, night workers always had that spaced out look in the morning. This confirmed in my mind that night work was clearly not designed for the human body to handle effectively. We're just not built to reverse our circadian rhythm (popularly referred to as the body clock).

She briefly introduced herself to me as Hannah, it was clear she was in a hurry to get home, so she quickly passed the keys over to Paul, and began reading through the printed out list in front of her. This was the first thing I noticed that was slightly different from working in the hospital. Usually we just stood in front of a big whiteboard full of names and the nurses used to read through them one by one.

Hannah kept reading through the list; nothing much had happened during the night, most people had slept well. One resident had spent a few moments crawling along the floor and shuffling along on his bottom, but had soon retired back to bed once he had got bored of this. This was common behaviour for him at night.

Once Hannah had finished the handover she was off, but not before the carers had quizzed her on how many residents she had woken up and dressed this morning. It would turn out that this was to be a constant source of anxiety for the day staff.

The less residents up in the morning meant more work for the carers during the day, i.e. they had more residents in bed that needed washing and dressing. Unfortunately it had started to become all about numbers. This was going directly against what I had learnt in university about person centred care and putting the patient first in everything you do.

This was the one and only concern of the day staff. The usual number of residents that were up, washed and dressed in the morning would be about six to nine. Any less than this number, then be prepared for the long stares and sarcastic comments behind your back, just out of hearing. Often the night staff would field this daily question in advance, reeling off the number of residents up, washed and dressed before the carers could bleat on about it.

To get the average of six to nine residents up meant the night staff would start getting people up at six in the morning. There were generally only one or two residents on the unit who had the capacity to make the decision if they wanted to get up or have a lie in. The rest were unable to comprehend or state a preference. Six in the morning seemed incredibly early (even during my training I thought eight in the morning was fairly early to be getting people up in the hospitals). Some nurses would even start getting people up from five thirty onwards. Dragging people out of bed, not for the sake of the resident's well-being, but to appease and make the day staff jobs easier. Interestingly, during my time as a student the hospital operated a very different policy. The night staff wouldn't be responsible for getting any patients up (only if they specifically requested it), so it was purely the day staff that would start getting them up from eight onwards.

Only two people worked on a unit at night, and there were at least five people working on a unit in the daytime. It was unfeasible to expect the same results from the night staff. The night staff were getting people up when they were at their most fatigued, towards the end of their shift. Day staff would be getting people up at the start of their shift. Basic maths. Pure and simple.

There was an incident where a new nurse who had only been on the unit for a matter of weeks undertook his first night shift. He did as he thought best and only got the residents up who were either wide awake or could have the capacity to state a choice. He got two residents up. The next morning the unit manager was on, and she was not impressed.

That afternoon an email went round to all the nurses stating that 'a minimum of six residents can always be got up each morning' and there was no excuses for not doing otherwise. Something that was inherently variable suddenly became fact, and from that day onwards, woe betide anyone who got any less than six up on a night shift. The story of the lowly crusading nurse who 'only got two people up' had become legend, a story that got passed down to all new nursing staff who were about to undertake their first night shift. He was considered something of a hero, someone who bucked the trend and fought for what the residents wanted.

A lot of the disagreements also stemmed from the fact that when the routine morning pad change round (pads resembled large adult nappies with varying absorbency) occurred around six in the morning, you would have to wake the residents in order to change their pad if they were incontinent. If they were awake then some of the managers argued that you might as well get them washed, dressed and up in the morning. A lot of the nurses argued that you were merely just disturbing them for a few minutes, and this did not constitute a justifiable reason to get them up. Most of the time they would simply go back to sleep once their pad had been changed.

Paul slowly pushed a piece of paper in front of the carers. The page stated 'daily work sheet', and seemed to be a paper that detailed exactly what jobs everyone would be assigned to during the day, and who would work with whom. It had spaces for who would be in charge of breakfast, lunch, and tea, morning and afternoon drinks, and who would be in charge of food and fluid charts. Paul started filling in this sheet as the carers chatted amongst themselves. The chart also detailed who would be on first and second break.

It was supposed to be the nurse in charge on that particular day who made the decisions as to who was doing what. The care assistants had very different ideas about this and there would be a constant power struggle involving this very simple bit of paper.

The carers would try to change the sheet, sometimes blatantly. Other times they would take the sheet away and pin it up on the board by the kitchen sink and start trading jobs between each other. If someone didn't feel like sorting out breakfast, they would often swap the tasks with each other, sometimes even swapping who they wanted to work with. If they were to alter the sheet in front of the nurse they would usually 'suggest' that someone work with someone else because they hadn't been on that side for a while, or other such inappropriate reasons. If the carers wanted things altering, they would get altered, despite the good intentions of the nurse in charge. It was a constant battle of wills and egos. The carers were clever, and would often try to manipulate and steer any younger nurse's decision making to their own advantage.

Other times the carers would simply swap over who they were working with halfway through the morning, thinking that the nurses wouldn't really notice. The nurses always noticed, but it was often a case of whether the nurse had the strength or assertiveness to say anything, or just keep a note of it and remember it for when a nurses meeting came up and raise the issue. All the management were aware of what was going on. And it was going to be an ongoing problem.

I went into the toilet around the corner from the nurse's station, with my new dark blue tunic. I normally hated tunics and had never worn the pristine white version from my university days, but luckily this one didn't feel too bad. I glance in the mirror and give myself a good long look. I recalled the film Wall Street and most particularly the scene with Charlie Sheen just before he is about to meet his mentor Gordon 'greed is good' Gecko. I recount the words in my head. 'Life comes down to just a few moments, and this is one of them'. I walk out of the bathroom, put my bag away in the store cupboard and start walking towards the lounge area again.

I see another resident walking around. He is fully dressed, with small amounts of white hair on either side of his bald head. He is incredibly stooped, almost staring directly at the floor, and he is salivating profusely. He is dressed in a dark brown cardigan, and has purple braces over a white checked shirt. He doesn't speak. He is simply walking up the corridor. As I pass him he tries to grab out at me with his hands. I slowly raise my hands towards his, and he gently holds them. He lets go a few seconds later, and carries on with his quest and walks down the corridor.

Jenny ushers me over.

'Right, if you come with me, it's time to sit everyone up first.'

I follow Jenny along the corridor. We walk into each of the residents' rooms one at a time, getting their tables ready, and sitting them up in the bed, putting people onto their backs, ready for their breakfast. We walk into a small old lady's room. She cries out.

'Hey! Where are my tablets?'

'Paul is doing the tablets, he won't be long.'

'Oh, I wish I had my tablets, my legs are killing me you know, where are they?'

'It's okay, he really won't be long, give him ten or fifteen minutes.'

Jilly rolls her eyes from left to right, and then smiles.

'Lovey, is it breakfast time already?'

'It is indeed Jilly!' Jenny replies.

'Can you put my teeth in please?'

Jenny walks into Jilly's bathroom, and gets a small box containing her false teeth. She hands the top set to Jilly, and she stares up at both Jilly and I.

'Have you got any stuff for them?'

Jenny seems to instantly produce a tube of Fixodent from her pocket, squeezes a small bit out onto the dentures, and hands them to Jilly.

'Thanks love, sticks them in better.'

'Wow! You're well prepared! Do you normally just carry Fixodent round in your pocket?' I enquire.

Jenny laughs and looks back at me.

'Jilly always wants a little bit. Always be prepared in this game, you will soon learn the tricks of the trade!'

We worked our way up the corridor, until everyone was ready and in the correct position for breakfast. We then walked back down to the lounge area. It was time to get breakfast under way.

The carers were rushing around gathering various trays and pouring out cups of tea into small plastic beakers. Jenny appeared to be in charge of dishing out the porridge and preparing the toast, whilst the others were pouring the tea and another would be sugaring them all. It was like one big production line. As I walked over to them a tray was immediately thrust towards me with two identical bowls of porridge and two beakers full of tea. The beakers were about half the size of a normal mug and had a plastic spout attached to the top of them. This was common with dementia. Many dementia patients have lost their swallow reflex, and will often not swallow properly or spill a lot of their drinks down them as they get confused or forget that they are holding something. A beaker simply helps reduce the chances of this and it becomes more efficient in making sure the residents are getting the fluid input they need each day.

Jenny was incredibly small and wore small black glasses. She had very short, curly hair. She wore a dark green cardigan over the top of her bright blue uniform. She had been in the care business for over fifteen years.

'Can you just feed Dwayne and Mark please, they're fine, Dwayne will eat with his eyes closed but don't worry about that, they're in rooms sixty one and sixty two, just past the nurse's station turn right.'

'Okay, no problem,' I say.

I was happy to get on with things and feel part of the team early on. Whilst I realised my main role here would be to nurse, I also appreciated that I needed to get to know the residents first hand, a phrase that was often called being 'on the floor'. I walked past the nurse's station and down the corridor. I had started to pick up a little bit of how the unit was split. The nurse's station formed the middle of the unit, to the right of the station were rooms sixty one to seventy. To the left of the station were rooms seventy one to eighty.

I approach room sixty one which is clearly labelled as Dwayne's room; I can hear some shouting coming from the room. I knock on the door and slowly enter. The room is dimly lit, with just a small lamp in the corner of the room; the main lights are switched off. Dwayne looks to be in his seventies with a completely bald, shiny head. He has a remarkable similarity to Roald Dahl's BFG (big friendly giant). I can immediately tell that Dwayne is incredibly tall, even though he is lying down. His large knees are thrust up beside his chin, and he is shouting with his eyes closed.

'No no no no no no no no no!' Dwayne shouts at the top of his voice. He appears to be responding to auditory hallucinations, as he keeps moving his head one way, then another.

'Please please please, Johnny Johnny Johnny Johnny!' he further shouts, still with his eyes remaining firmly shut.

I step inside further until I am right next to Dwayne.

'Hi Dwayne, I'm Jack, I have just got some breakfast for you, some porridge and a nice cup of tea.'

Dwayne keeps his eyes firmly shut but responds to me.

'Yes alright then,' Dwayne replies in a soft voice.

I begin slowly spoon feeding Dwayne some of his porridge. He keeps taking the food off me as quickly as I can deliver it, still with his eyes firmly shut. After a brief minute his porridge is consumed, and I give him the cup of tea, which he takes from me and with a bit of gentle prompting he is able to drink most of it himself. Throughout the whole process Dwayne has not opened his eyes at all. As soon as I place the bowl of porridge and beaker of tea back on the tray Dwayne begins to shout again, this time raising his hands forward and pointing towards the wall in front of him.

'Johnny, Johnny no no no no no!'

He continues using his fists to gesture towards the wall, all the while keeping his eyes firmly shut. I step outside his room and continue to the opposite room.

Mark was completely bed-bound, having lost the ability to walk a long time ago. He would be hoisted into the chair in his room for a minimum of two hours per day so his wife could spend some time sat next to him. These two hours, although the minimum, helped to relieve pressure sore areas that he would frequently get on his body. This was common practice with the elderly, as pressure sore areas were very frequent.

An elderly person's skin is much more fragile than our own and even their own weight on certain areas of their body (most commonly their sacral area –

the lower part of your back) can cause the skin to break down. If you don't relieve the pressure as much as possible by turning the resident every two to four hours, then these pressure areas would become red and sore and eventually cause very nasty pressure sores that invite further infection. Most bed bound residents would have specific turn charts, and it was the care assistant's role to ensure these were adhered to.

Mark did not speak any more. He could give you some basic gestures and sometimes would smile and laugh at you, but his use of speech went a long time ago. His wife, Deirdre, visited every single lunchtime without fail, and stayed with Mark till about seven each evening, giving him support and company. Mark had been here almost two years, and hadn't changed much in his appearance. He continued to eat and drink well most days; his wife was very supportive to the nursing team and always trusted the judgement of the staff.

Mark had deep set dark brown eyes, and jet black hair. He smiled at me as I walked in. He was holding a small brown stuffed dog toy in his right hand. This toy had varying purposes, as Mark had the tendency to grab hold of your hand or uniform and hold it very tightly without letting go. The toy dog helped alleviate the frequency of this and helped the staff get on with their daily duties. Feeding Mark was no problem at all. At times he would try and grab hold of the beaker full of tea and try to drink it himself. I let him do this to the best of his ability. Engaging and allowing the residents to do as much as they can for as long as they can was still in my mind from my university training, and we should always be trying to ensure that this continues for as long as possible.

As I looked around Mark's room I saw many pictures on the walls from his younger days. There was a picture of him in full Army regalia, and another with him hugging his wife in what looked to be their garden. This was often the saddest thing working in mental health; seeing people how they were before their illness took hold, and seeing them in their home environments with friends and family.

After I had fed Mark, I returned to the lounge area where most of the care assistants were busying themselves around the Bain Marie, a large metal construction on wheels which kept all the food piping hot and had various drawers, shelves and containers within it, keeping all the food separate.

There was an unwritten rule in this home that once all the residents had been fed in the morning, the staff were allowed to have an egg or bacon sandwich, as they were only going to go to waste and be thrown away. The kitchen staff argued that they needed specific details of what food was being left, so they can adjust their amounts accordingly on a daily basis. If the staff are taking this food, then they won't have an accurate enough picture, and won't be able to order and cook the correct amount of bacon, egg and porridge for the residents each morning.

Daily changes in residents eating habits will occur anyway, so by its very nature the amount of food being provided will always be a best guess. The management still consider 'taking off the trolley' after morning feeding times as theft. Usually it would depend on which staff members were on shift, and if the management were about and walking around the unit of a morning. The jury was still out, but many of the care assistants would take the odd bit of toast or bowl of porridge and eat it discreetly.

There were a number of smokers within the care assistant community. A few of the carers would take the Bain Marie out of the lounge area (as it was still hot, and posed a risk to mobile residents) and pop it outside the unit ready to be picked up and restocked. The other carers would then take the trolley down to the kitchen area. The other trolley was just a small grey trolley with wheels on it, which housed all the dirty beakers and plates and bowls that needed cleaning up. The carers who took the trolley down to the kitchen would take the opportunity to have a quick cigarette break at the smoking shelter before returning back onto the unit ready to start getting people up and out of bed.

Forget management, and forget chain of command, emails and meetings. The smoking shelter was the epicentre of all information, gossip and rumour. If anything was happening within the business, it arrived at the smoking shelter first, before being passed by word of mouth throughout the rest of the building. The smoking shelter was a small shed situated right next to the laundry, and had a small area with cheap seating. Chairs that would have usually been destined for the skip were all arranged in a row underneath the shelter, and this is where most of the care assistants went for breaks. All news of pregnancies or major life changing news would be broken here. Not many nurses frequented the shelter, but if they did, they would probably be far more informed about what was going on than most upper management.

All cigarette breaks outside of normal break times were unofficial. Whilst the smokers went off for a quick smoke, the rest of the carers left on the unit would start getting people up. This started a rift and some unrest, as the non smokers argued they were working more than the smokers. Over the course of a day the smokers could clock up an extra thirty minutes in 'fag breaks' over the non smokers. Eventually this all came to a head, and through various management meetings this was deemed an improper use of staff time so early in the morning. Most would abide by this rule, but the stronger characters would still utilise their assertiveness by using the trolley as an excuse to leave the unit, even sometimes saying to the nurse in charge of the unit 'You know what we are doing' with a sly wink and nod, putting the responsibility on the nurse in charge, but still going ahead and having a sneaky cigarette, even though they knew they were breaking the rules.

Paul had opened up the medicine trolley and was starting to do the medication. The medicine trolley was kept locked away at all other times. Paul was wheeling it gently up the corridor and moving it on after dispensing individual medication to the relevant resident.

'How's it going matey?' he enquired.

'Yeah not bad, getting into it slowly,' I say.

'You will be fine, don't worry, we will show you the ropes. I'll get you in the office later and we can go through some of the paperwork.'

'Great, yeah, no worries,' I reply. I wasn't in a huge rush to get into the office, but I realised the importance of understanding the paperwork for when I was ultimately in charge.

Paul had a great manner about him and as he went into each resident's room he would shout out 'Good Morning', and give the residents a little bit of small talk, and try to make them smile. At all times he was telling the residents what he was doing and that he had their 'medication' or 'tablets' for them. It was always important to stress this, even if you thought the residents no longer had any comprehension of what you were giving them. This was best practice, and Paul was adhering to this at all times. Paul would sing to himself as he strolled up and down the corridor wheeling his trolley.

'Right matey, if you work with Emma this morning and just get people up, washed and dressed, then we can start doing some office work after that, okay?'

'Yeah, sure, no problem,' I say.

Emma was an incredibly tall girl, who overshot me by a good few feet (and I was about 5ft 10 inches). She had straight brown hair tied up into a bunch behind her and small Jasper Conran designer glasses. She looked to be in her early twenties, and appeared very bubbly and full of smiles. Emma immediately directed me to where the aprons were, where we both put on blue plastic aprons.

'Right, if we go and get Vancy up first then see who else is about, as she is often awake at this time,' Emma stated very assertively.

'Sure thing,' I say.

Procedure should always be to work in pairs, and if you were getting up female patients, to have either two females, or a female and a male. Never males only, as it was felt it was not appropriate or fair to the resident's dignity, or preference. There had been a complaint many months ago from a resident who had been awoken by a single male. The resident had enough capacity to retain this information, and tell her daughter that she wasn't happy with a male getting her up in the morning and helping her to get washed and dressed. The daughter filed a complaint with the unit, and from then on, they have had to be far more vigilant and pro active when pairing up people to work with females. As a male you are at a disadvantage in this respect, and have to pay more attention to areas like this and not put yourself in a position where you could jeopardise your career by not being careful and safe, always putting the resident's dignity first.

I had come under considerable fire in my student days from this very argument about male and females. As a student nurse, working on a learning disabilities placement, I was frequently called upon to wash and shower females on my own. I had gone along with this initially, trying to be a good and hard working student, but I had felt uncomfortable from the offset. I had made my feelings known to the management and they had come back to me with the NMC guide on chaperoning.

Chaperoning

'Nurses and midwives have a professional duty to assist people in their care in making decisions regarding their treatment or care, by providing them with sufficient information. Nurses and midwives must ensure that the person in their care has been provided with - and understands - a full explanation of the procedure or examination to be carried out.'

'Theoretically, there is no difference between situations where a male nurse or midwife is caring for a woman or where a female nurse or midwife is caring for a man. The issue to be considered in both cases is whether the situation is acceptable to that person and, perhaps, those close to them.'

'Where intimate procedures or examinations are required, nurses and midwives should ensure that they are aware of any cultural, religious beliefs or restrictions the person in their care may have, which prohibits this being done by a member of the opposite sex. Any preferences and/or objections to care management

> should be identified as early as possible to eliminate the potential of causing any unnecessary offence. The individual requirements of the person should be respected and the preference documented in the appropriate records.'
>
> > 'Nurses and midwives are also advised to ensure they are familiar with local policies regarding chaperoning.'
>
> **Nursing and Midwifery Council, (2008) - guidelines on chaperoning**

I had a professional duty to wash and care for people, however there were many female care assistants working in this particular placement. The person in question could not tell me whether she thought the situation was acceptable as she had lost the ability to speak. The manager had told me that the female in question would 'easily be able to indicate that she wasn't happy with me being there by non verbal indicators'. I still wasn't happy with the situation, so I dug my heels in and complained. Luckily there was a kind female nurse working there who agreed with my principles. She said I was right to refuse.

I continued to refuse to wash and dress female residents on my own, and this had caused considerable annoyance and agitation amongst the female carers. Many an argument ensued, most notably being that the female carers had to wash both sexes. I was considered lazy because I only wanted to wash same sex individuals.

I understood the duty of care and in this instance there were plenty of staff on duty to complement the mix adequately and provide a duty of care to all patients involved with a suitable mix of female and male carers. I thought that the reason I was pushed into attending to female patients on my own was the argument of saving time and getting the student out of the way. As a result, when it became time for my final assessment and sign off I was marked down because of my poor personal care skills. This didn't detract at all from my eventual qualification, but it served as a reminder as to how some clinical areas and staff will certainly try to 'bully' students into doing things they don't want to do. It had taught me a valuable lesson in standing up for what I believed in.

In the home there would be a continual battle about who should work in pairs and others who would take it upon themselves to get people up on their own. Sometimes there may be residents that can be easily washed and dressed by someone on their own, but from a safety point of view this was still unsafe practice. The biggest argument was that some carers were simply able to work faster and more efficiently on their own, and preferred it. Working in pairs could be slower, but then this was not a race, it was twenty four hour care. By working in pairs you were giving that resident extra attention and providing more secure quality care. In the staff contract, it clearly stated the following:

'At no time whilst undertaking your duties within our Home must you attempt to lift or support *any* patient on your own. All moving of patients must be carried out by a minimum of two members of staff or by the use of the patient moving and handling equipment, which has been provided for the purpose. You have a responsibility for your own health and safety and that of your colleagues and we take moving and handling issues extremely seriously. If you feel you are being put in an uncomfortable situation where either you or a service user is being placed at risk please report the matter immediately to a senior member of staff.'

It was there in black and white, but still people wouldn't adhere to this at times.

Emma showed me the way down to Vancy's room. The carers usually split equally and one team would cover one side, and the other team the other side. This would also cause problems at times, when one team had finished their 'side' first; they would often go on their allotted break time, rather than helping out the other side in getting the rest of the residents up. Numerous attempts at changing the daily work sheet to avoid this never seemed to work either.

Attempts at changing the numbered sides (which corresponded to the room numbers) to indicate 'red' or 'blue' sides hadn't been successful either. The carers just decided which side each colour was, and it was back to square one. The sides would change on a daily basis depending on what side the carers wished to work on.

At one point the sheet even read 'one side' and 'the other', but this also didn't work. The carers would always find a way, and their way always seemed to win out in the end, despite numerous interventions. They seemed to become highly territorial about their protected sides of the unit, and this was always a bone of contention between other carers, right down to whether someone needed changing in the evening.

If a resident who needed changing was on one carer's 'side' of the unit, that carer was expected to go and change the resident. It would be a continual battle to try and move the carers back into a more holistic and person centred approach, trying to look at the person and their individual preferences. Team work seemed to be distinctly lacking, and carers would often use their 'sides' to their advantage.

Sadly it was becoming far too task orientated, treating each stage of the day as a specific task which was time limited. It didn't seem to matter how many times you reiterated the point that dementia was variable, and that people simply wouldn't fit neatly into little boxes. Carers would find a way to fit these people into boxes, no matter what, despite what the Government or the latest reports said. Living in the 'real world' was still a far cry from the ideals set out by legislation, backed up with evidence based research.

How can we improve dementia care?
June Andrews, director of Dementia Services Development Centre, offers the following advice. I offer my own experiences after each sub heading:

- **'Ask the four simple questions that will tell you if your patient is cognitively impaired':**
  What is your name?
  What day is it?
  When were you born?
  What is this place?

If one of our residents is in our home, they will not necessarily have any means to find out what day it is other than the whiteboard in the lounge area which has a very faint marker pen stating what day it actually is, which barely any member of staff can read, let alone a resident. Other than that, they are dependent on either a paper (which most residents do not have) or a member of staff telling them what day it is (which doesn't always happen).

- **'Remember that undiagnosed and untreated pain is the most common cause of disturbing behaviour in dementia. Most older people in hospital have pain, so check that it has been assessed. If not, tell someone.'**

A lot of residents will often be on regular paracetamol, or have a matrifen pain relief patch. This is where you have to really use your observational skills, and for less obvious pain, there are various pain assessment tools available that you can try to utilise.

- **'Introduce yourself every time you see people with dementia.'**

I would always greet my residents, particularly residents who would often cover many miles up and down the corridor, and each and every time they glanced in my direction I would say hello, and sometimes they would respond. Initially I felt a bit strange continually saying hello to people (this could happen over a dozen times a day at times), but once you get a real understanding of dementia, you realise the importance of this greeting.

- **'Find out their background. A retired admiral can be comforted in a slightly different way from a retired cook. One can respect them equally, but addressing them in the same manner could be uncomfortable for both.'**

The more you knew about someone, the more you could relate. I remember my student days when I was working with a young lad with depression who used to live in the same area I grew up in. I was instantly able to build a rapport, and discuss local pubs and bars we had both frequented. This is often the 'bare bones' of building rapport, having life experience. It can massively help to gain that trust, and it's often a considerable advantage. Universities also take into account life experience when looking at potential applicants to mental health nursing courses.

- **'When with patients, think only about how to make them comfortable. Nothing else matters'**

If you don't agree with this, then you shouldn't be in nursing.

- **'It is better to distract and comfort confused people, rather than arguing or trying to prove that they are wrong.'**

Distraction always worked well for me. At times I would offer people to help me do the laundry, or stock towels in residents' rooms. Anything to distract and try to get them focused. It's not always easy, but you had to think outside of the box at times, and be quite random in your own thinking; whatever distracts can be a massive help.

Sometimes doing a medication round I would have various residents follow me into other residents' rooms. I took on the role of a 'mentor' and explained to them who I was administering medication to next. Some would find this very interesting and keep following me round, but the important factor was that they were not distressed and I had kept their attention.

- **'Use every opportunity for appropriate touch'**

I cannot count the times I offered a hand to an elderly gentleman or lady to shake in greeting. It was one of the most basic non verbal gestures, and often had results. It was all part of gaining trust and rapport. Communication covered all aspects, and that included your body language. Many a resident has given me a nod, a sly wink, and complete genuine appreciation or recognition.

Sometimes the most basic gestures were the most effective. Holding someone's hand also gave you the most powerful resonance and completeness at times. Listening to someone tell their story whilst you hold their hand, in their greatest hour of need, was often more effective than anything medication could offer.

- **'Do not worry about repeating yourself when talking to patients, and be sure to listen attentively to their tales, even if they repeat them. This is a part of care, not an annoying side issue.'**

Hard to get used to at first, but you have to appreciate the extent of some residents' memory loss. I have had residents ask me where the toilet is, or where the exit is, and then ask me the same question ten seconds later. Sometimes you feel like they are on a continual loop. But you cannot falter; you have to remain attentive and try to understand.

- **'Rely as much as you can on the carer, whether it is the care home care assistant or a visiting family member. They know short cuts to all of the above.'**

You should never underestimate your team of carers. Despite the bickering or politics that may go on in your place of work, they are your 'ground force' that are mapping your residents, day in, day out. They know the nuances and the tricks for every possible outcome. They know if your residents take a small spoon rather than a large one for example.

They know that they require a drink after their meal is given, because otherwise they will tip their drink all over the table. They know how to dress each resident, if they should be standing, or sat on the toilet. Don't underestimate what your team of carers understand about your residents. They do this job day in, day out. Use their wealth of knowledge to help you build the ultimate map of your resident, which in turn will mean the best possible care for them.

- **'Use your imagination. Busy work with a duster or a pile of paperwork can occupy people with dementia for hours and prevent them wandering or, worse, having an accident.'**

I would often ask residents to join me in doing the laundry, or stocking rooms with towels. I would have residents sat in the nursing station and I would offer them pieces of paper, offer them cups of tea, glasses of wine or whisky if appropriate whilst talking to them as a friend.

> I would continually be striving to offer any sense of distraction no matter where I was. You have to think outside of the box. These were real people. Imagine yourself with nothing to do, day in, day out; everyone needs a sense of purpose. Something to occupy your mind.
>
> As a student I would often utilise whatever was in the ward's storage cupboards, be that a few blocks of Lego or playing cards, or dominoes. It would often have a considerable impact on residents. You just had to keep on trying, no matter how stupid it might feel.
>
> I had many residents gathered around a table once, as a student, with piles of Lego bricks, and they started to build what they liked. They were actively engaged. I had held their attention. Better that than falling over, or being completely bored and becoming more and more agitated.
>
> **All Imaginative Care dementia tips taken from Andrews, (2010)**

We got down to Vancy's room. The door was already open, and immediately I could tell that the room was very hot and musty, with a peculiar smell. Some carers would define this smell as the 'smell of death'. Vancy was fully awake, bolt upright in her bed.

Vancy was ninety five years of age, with a very withered and elongated face, but with bright white styled hair. Her eyes were incredibly sunken, and she had a large amount of loose skin under each one. Her frail hands were covered in age spots. She turned towards me, and spoke out.

'Help me, help me, help, help, help, I'm frightened. I am you know!' Vancy was not appearing to be able to express why she was frightened. Just that she was.

Emma turned towards me. 'It's okay, we seem to have variable days with Vancy, she is either quite manic and anxious one day, or completely asleep and settled on another.'

Vancy was indeed very changeable. Her dementia had been like this for a long while, so much so that the consultants and GP had no further ideas on what to do regarding her medication. She was currently written up for Lorazepam up to 4mg a day (1mg, four times a day). Lorazepam was known as a benzodiazepine, usually indicated for short term relief of severe anxiety. Long term use should be avoided. Unfortunately Vancy had been on these particular drugs for a very long time.

The nursing team and doctors were working towards her best interests and had to weigh up the potential side effects against the potential relief that Vancy would be getting by having these particular drugs. There were numerous side effects, as with all medications, including a paradoxical increase in aggression, drowsiness, light headedness and confusion being the most common.

Sadly this medication didn't seem to be working as well as it should be. The elderly should actually only be given half the maximum dose that you would normally give to adults, meaning that Vancy should only be given a maximum of 2mg. However the doctors and professional team had decided that this was their best shot in trying to alleviate her anxiety, and hence she was put on the maximum dose of 4mg. The other problem with this type of drug is that eventually the body will build up a resistance to it, and as a result the drug becomes less effective over time. This was the case with Vancy, and as Emma had described, they were at a bit of a crossroads. One day it would either knock Vancy flat, and other days it wouldn't seem to touch her at all, and she would be in the state she was this morning, anxious and unable to comprehend or rationalise her feelings in any way at all.

> **How does dementia medication work?**
>
> 'There are two main types of drugs that are used to treat Alzheimer's disease. They are known as acetyl cholinesterase inhibitors. Research shows that the brains of people with Alzheimer's disease show a loss of nerve cells that use a chemical called acetylcholine as a chemical messenger. The loss of these nerve cells relates to how severe an impairment people experience.'
>
> - **Aricept** (Donepezil Hydrochloride) – the first drug to be licensed in the UK specifically for Alzheimer's disease.
>
> - **Exelon** (Rivastigmine) – the second drug licensed in the UK specifically for Alzheimer's disease.
>
> - **Reminyl** (Galantamine) – Originally derived from the bulbs of snowdrops and narcissi, the third drug licensed in the UK specifically for Alzheimer's disease.
>
> - **Ebixa** (Memantine) – the newest of the Alzheimer's drugs.

> 'Aricept, Exelon and Reminyl prevent an enzyme known as acetyl cholinesterase from breaking down acetylcholine in the brain. Increased concentrations of acetylcholine lead to increased communication between the nerve cells that use acetylcholine as a chemical messenger, which may improve or stabilise temporarily the symptoms of Alzheimer's disease.'
>
> 'Ebixa is slightly different, and complex. It blocks a chemical messenger known as glutamate. Glutamate is released in excessive amounts when brain cells are damaged by Alzheimer's disease.'
>
> 'This causes the brain cells to be damaged further. Ebixa acts to protect these brain cells by blocking excess glutamate.'
>
> 'It is important to remember that all dementia drugs are designed to slow down the progression of the disease, and maintain quality of life for as long as possible. There is no current cure for dementia.'
>
> **Alzheimer's Society, (2011)**

I could not begin to describe how many times Vancy shouted out the words help in such quick succession. At one point she was actually close to frothing at the mouth.

'Help me, help, help, help, help, I'm frightened, help, help, help, help!' she shouted, before pausing for a second.

'Help!' A second pause.

'Help! Please!'

'Hellllllllpppppp.' She was shouting so much her voice almost broke in pitch. Emma and I managed to gradually stand her up and begin dressing her.

Vancy was sometimes able to help a little with getting herself dressed, but only very slightly, maybe by putting the odd arm through her cardigan or lifting her feet as you put her socks on. Today she wasn't able to help at all.

We both stand her up and slowly walk her to the toilet. We sit her down and Emma begins to wash her.

Emma pulls the light cord. Nothing happens.

'Oh no, power's gone again'

'Power?'

'It does this now and again, the last four rooms lose power, something trips the switch, and they just have to flick the switch back on. They have had numerous engineers in here, and the best they can come up with is to just keep trying various switches, and try to monitor what exactly is causing the electricity to fail.'

Emma pokes her head outside Vancy's room and shouts up the corridor.

'Paul! Electricity out again!'

A faint shout from Paul can be heard from down the corridor.

'Okay!'

Emma walks into Vancy's bathroom, and waits a few moments. She tries the pull cord again, and the light comes on.

'Absolutely ridiculous, this place, at times'

I remember my very first student placement and being so terrified about washing and dressing people, but now it seemed second nature, although I was still a little apprehensive due to it being such a new environment. Vancy was trying to get up off the seat a few times, but with gradual reassurance and talking to her, she settled, but only for brief pockets of time. We were careful to explain what we were doing at each step of the process. It didn't always seem to work, but it was best practice.

Vancy was eventually washed and dressed, so we gradually walk her out of her bathroom and sit her down in her wheelchair, and I push her into the lounge area. We then stand her up gently and sit her back down into the chair; Emma gets her a cup of tea, and pushes it in front of her.

'There you go Vancy, here's a cup of tea for you' Emma says.

Vancy looked up at Emma with her dull sunken eyes.

'Thank you love.' For a brief second Vancy had almost forgotten how anxious she was, and took the beaker of tea and lifted it up to her mouth and began taking small gulps of it.

In her day Vancy had been a professional singer, singing and playing the piano at many stage and theatre productions up and down the country. Her voice was still powerful today, sadly only being able to shout out cries for help. Emma and I leave Vancy to her beaker of tea and grab a fresh blue apron.

As I walked up the corridor, I could hear Vancy faintly talking to herself, very softly, not agitated like before, or anxious, but just quietly to herself.

'Help me, please help me.'

'Help.'

'Help.....'

'Help.'

9–10 a.m.

Emma and I put on our blue plastic aprons. Sharon and Katie are walking down towards us from the opposite end of the corridor. Sharon was an 'old school' carer, just passed her sixtieth birthday, and she was a complete work horse. She had bleached blond hair dragged back into a pony tail very tightly. She was short in stature, but with a loud and commanding voice. Sharon would often bark her orders out and keep the unit on an even keel.

Originally from Sheffield, Sharon had been working for the company since its inception. She had worked on all the units in her time, and she knew all the tricks of the trade. She would often take the young carers under her wing and train them her way. For a sixty year old she could run rings around most of the carers on the unit, quick to break in new members of staff, or send them running to the job centre for a change of career. Her husband had been very ill for a number of years with lung cancer. She often described coming to work as a break, and enjoyed everyone's company, and used her time here to give herself a change of scenery from her life back home. She worked a thirty hour week.

Sharon could verbally reduce you to tears within a few seconds if she wished, but equally she could be the nicest and most supportive carer there was. You just had to get on the right side of her. A lot of the carers would often complain that Sharon would order them around, and a few had stood up to her, but it would often end in tears. Sharon was a law unto herself at times, but the management trusted her, respected her, and were not in a hurry to get rid of her.

Sharon had come under particular fire of late, due to her poor attendance, and letting her fellow team members down at the last minute. In the past few months she had clocked up a total of seventeen non attendances, due either to sickness, or family issues. She would usually ring up very close to the date that she was due to be in, sometimes that morning. Everyone was entitled to be ill, but Sharon was starting to be quite predictable on her non attendance, most notably during the weekend shifts, where the staffing levels were needed the most. She had been hauled into the management office more times than most carers had hot dinners. She just didn't care. She had received letters from the management telling her that she was being formally disciplined, and that it was a form of gross misconduct. But Sharon simply sat in the office each time, and let the manager give her a lecture on the fact that she was not attending as much as she should be. On her last visit she had simply just said 'Just do what you have to.'

The management were very reluctant to do anything about it. The only thing the management and Sharon had agreed upon was to reduce her hours by six, from thirty to twenty four. Sharon would be committing to just two days a week, rather than two and a half days a week. It had struck the other carers that Sharon probably didn't really need the money much; it was more about spending time away from her difficult family life. This probably gave Sharon a lot more power than most of the other carers who needed the job, and couldn't afford to drop hours, or lose money from ringing in sick. Sharon would utilise her more powerful position over the other carers, and cleverly control them in an insidious manner. She may not act like she knew what she was doing, but beneath the surface, there was a clever and calculating manipulator of behaviour and influence. And it got results.

Katie was a very slender girl with dark brown glasses and dark brown hair tied into a pony tail. She couldn't have been more than twenty years of age. Katie was Jennifer's (the acting manager's) daughter. She was due to start her nurse training next year, and had been here since the home had opened. When her mother was given the opportunity to be acting manager, the carers were all rather sceptical about how this would affect their relationship with Katie. Jennifer was often quick to point out that she would never discuss business with Katie, and everything was confidential outside of work. Many staff would think that you couldn't trust Katie with any sort of complaints or general gossip about the home as it would get straight back to her mother. This put everyone in quite a difficult situation. Some people felt that Katie was like a 'spy' sent to infiltrate and report back anything that she thought was wrong to her mother at every available opportunity. Katie would frequently deny this and laugh off such preposterous allegations.

Katie was a hard worker, and very helpful towards the nursing staff, and very keen to get stuck in. Often the carers would feel she was a bit too keen and frequently not work as a team player and work under her own steam, getting residents up washed and dressed on her own. One shift there was Paul and two other male members of staff, a rarity in healthcare. Male members of staff were often in the minority. Paul said it was a breath of fresh air, and nice to work with a few other males, and had a fantastic shift. There would never be three males working on the same unit after that day though. Katie was furious, silently seething on the day of the shift, going off to do things on her own, but not asking any of the males for any help. She said that the male members of staff were simply just sitting around doing paperwork. The next day she went straight to her mother, and said to not put three male members of staff on again. The verdict? She didn't. Paul never worked with the two male members of staff ever since Katie had complained.

Male nurses

'One third of the almost 100,000 nurses who have a mental health qualification are men. Professor Sigsworth reluctantly sees some truth in the dominant thinking of the 1980's that the status of nursing would rise if it attracted more men, and that if nursing is seen as women's work, society tends to devalue it.'

'Several male nurses have contacted Nursing Standard to point out the anomalies around the gender divide in nursing. While female patients feel comfortable requesting a female nurse, male patients may not feel as at ease asking for a male nurse to care for them, they point out. It is often wrongly assumed that male patients will not mind.'

'Men are twice as likely to have posts in the higher nursing grades. They are also twice as likely to expect to move to a better job in the near future even though their female colleagues had better post – basic nursing qualifications and were just as career orientated.'

Nursing Standard, (2010)

During my practice I am always very careful when being asked to help dress a female resident (or indeed an intimate nursing procedure) that I am with another female carer, or ask a female nurse to complete a procedure.

> I would always ask if the resident minds me being in the room, and very clear to explain what needs to be done. It is all too easy sometimes to be pushed into getting people up on your own due to staffing issues. Whilst you have a duty of care, when there is a choice available on staff mix, then you should always offer that choice to your resident, and ask them if they are okay with you helping them. Giving them the courtesy and dignity helps to enforce their own wellbeing.
>
> Never assume just because a resident cannot speak or indicate a preference, that their values and choices should be ignored. They still have a right for good quality and dignified care.

Paul had come under considerable fire when being asked by other units to lend staff members out. If the unit was fully staffed with five members of staff, and another unit understaffed, it would often mean that a staff member would have to go across to another unit to help out, either for a morning, afternoon, or sometimes an entire day. Most staff were quite territorial and preferred to stay put on their unit, particularly if the other units who needed the help were the more general side of nursing. One morning, Paul had to send someone across. He decided to send Katie across. He confronted Katie. But this morning Katie had had enough. She refused to go across, because she claimed she was always the one to go over and help out, and Paul should send someone else.

Paul had only recently been appointed onto the unit, and he did not like being undermined. Jennifer had said it was his choice who to send, and he chose to send Katie. Katie left for her lunch break, and upon returning, waited patiently on the unit with another carer.

Whilst Paul was in the office the phone rang. Jennifer was on the other end of the phone.

'Paul, who is going across to Gerald unit today?'

'I've told Katie to go across.'

'No, send Emma across, okay, thank you.'

Jennifer had abruptly put the phone down. Paul walked out of the nursing station. Katie was still sat down at the table, almost smugly. Paul knew exactly what she had done; she had gone and complained to her mother about always going across. Paul had to send Emma. His power of authority had been undermined within a few moments. Paul had always thought he should have the final say as the nurse in charge.

People would often be moved from unit to unit, usually without even being asked. The rotas were prepared on a monthly basis. One day you could be checking your rota and suddenly realise that your name was not on the list. The reason why would be because it would be down on another rota, on another unit. The main reason for this would be that it 'improved skills' by moving carers and nurses around.

In cases of dementia, it would be a good idea to promote familiarity. Seeing the same faces, on a daily basis, helps build rapport and trust with residents. A good team of carers who support each other and get on well is far more productive than one that continually feels de-motivated, and is always being moved around to units in which they don't feel comfortable. When carers are moved frequently without being consulted about their own opinion, this usually forces them to either put up with it or simply hand in their resignation. There were plenty of other nursing homes where they could gain employment, and many moved on if they were not happy.

> **Support and Supervision**
> The latest Care Quality Commission report had flagged up only one area that needed addressing, and that was the role of supervision. We as nurses are required to have clinical supervision at least once every six weeks. I had been lucky, and continued to do this with a lecturer at the university where I had trained. Since joining the company I had never been offered supervision, until the commission had done their report. Almost immediately, the forms came flooding into the office and carers had to assign themselves to a nurse with whom they would feel comfortable talking about any areas of their work and be supported in these areas.
>
> Most of the carers saw this as a huge hindrance. A few of the carers who were studying their NVQ's found it very useful, as they had to provide evidence of supervision in order to pass the NVQ. The other carers really didn't see how supervision was going to work, as you needed at least a good hour off the unit to properly discuss anything. A few names went down, and a few were assigned to me. Nevertheless, to this day, I have only done one proper supervision with a carer, who needed it for her NVQ profile of evidence. The rest of the carers either tore up their supervision contracts or didn't fill them in. I imagine that this is an area that will once again be flagged up. There was no real promise of any protected time in which to do the supervision, and supervision often had to be rescheduled if there was an emergency or lots of ill residents on the unit who required more focused attention.

The carers would probably be more amenable if management had actually asked them if they would mind moving. Most of the carers were well trained, and most were being put in for their National Vocational Qualifications (NVQ) levels two and three.

Once a carer had achieved NVQ two, they would get a pound more an hour pay rise. Once up to a NVQ three, then they would receive no extra pay rise at all. Most NVQ three carers would then leave to find employment elsewhere that would suitably recognise their recent achievements. This appeared to be a common pattern, and one that didn't appear to be changing any time soon.

Sharon comes up to me and starts to bark her orders out at me in her thick northern accent, very loudly and firmly. She drops in the word 'baby' after most sentences. Sounding like 'beehhh beee.'

'Alright baby, Edward needs doing next okay? Then we will need to bath little Joanna, okay baby? Edward will need the stand aid just to transfer him up off the bed and into his chair. Just sit him in his chair in his room, and he can have his lunch there.'

'Sure, which room's Edward in?' I say.

'Room seventy three baby, just up here and to the left.'

Emma and I walk into Edward's room. Edward is an eighty three year old gentleman with dementia, chronic kidney disease, insulin dependent diabetic, recently diagnosed with bowel cancer. There had been considerable debate about whether Edward should be told of his diagnosis, or even if he would comprehend or understand what this meant.

There is a great wealth of information and evidence to support the telling of patient's news such as this and most evidence points towards the fact that people should be entitled to know and deserve to be told. You always need to weigh up the pros and cons of any such decision as some news could clearly have a devastating and massive impact on someone's well being and mind set.

Initially the unit manager had decided to tell Edward of his bowel cancer, and was very clear and straightforward about what this would mean. Afterwards Edward had turned towards the manager and said 'I wish you hadn't told me that now', and was quite understandably dejected and down. A few days later it was hard to tell if Edward had retained this information.

Edward had been a farmer all his life, enjoying working for himself buying and selling pigs and chickens, and had retired with his wife to spend a happy retirement. He had sold the farm off and moved into a two bed semi to spend his 'golden years' in comfort. Within a year of retiring to his new household he had been diagnosed with dementia. Initially his wife tried to cope with his illness at home; this was common. Sadly dementia progresses and people's needs become greater and much harder for someone's partner to be able to cope with them at home. After a spell in the local psychiatric hospital for assessment and treatment, Edward eventually had a place here at the home where he has remained for the past year.

As Edward's dementia had progressed, some of the female carers had started to complain that Edward was becoming a little too familiar with some of them, outstretching his hand to touch their breasts or bottom.

Edward was completely bed bound and due to his diabetes and varying blood sugar levels was incredibly tired for most of the day, often sleeping for many hours. The carers passed this information on to the nurse in charge on the shift, and ultimately to the unit manager.

During ward round, the nurse on shift at the time discussed with the doctors any changes or updates on the residents' presentation. It was decided by both the nurse and the doctor that Edward needed to be put onto another drug to curb his sexual inappropriateness.

Benperidol was their drug of choice. Edward was started off immediately on a dose of 0.25mg. Benperidol was a class of antipsychotic medication, for specific 'control of deviant antisocial sexual behaviour'. This drug was often used for sexual offenders, including paedophiles. Edward could not walk and was very slow in his movement. The doctor at the time was overheard saying 'We also need to keep the carers happy don't we?' and that he was 'on the lowest dose'.

Originally the doctor wanted to put Edward on two tablets each evening, but the nursing team decided only one was initially necessary. The most notable side effect from this drug was likely to be tardive dyskenisia (involuntary writhing movements of the facial muscles and tongue), extra pyramidal symptoms (various movement disorders), hypotension, drowsiness, cardiovascular changes and depression.

Edward immediately began to experience what appeared to be direct side effects of the drug, considerably leaning to one side during meal times and even more drowsiness. Edward seemed okay in himself and in his general mood. When Paul had asked the unit manager how long Edward was going to be on the drug, she had coldly replied 'Forever'.

There is no widely agreed definition of when a behaviour becomes abnormal, the decision is usually based either on a judgement of what is normal for a person in a particular situation. In this case the unit manager who was female decided that it would be a better course of action to suggest the commencement of Benperidol so as not to upset or make the care assistants' jobs more difficult when getting Edward up in the morning.

As nurses we are responsible for making decisions based upon the best interests of our patient, and when considerable risks to either themselves or others become apparent we need to be able to act upon this in a professional and responsible manner. It is a difficult decision to add to the already large mix of medication that Edward was taking, and potentially further risking his health and life span by adding this drug. Paul had fought to defend the decision, but the wave of resentment from the carers had simply been too much.

I walk into the room just behind Emma. Emma shouts out.

'Oh god.'

I immediately have a wave of anxiety rush over me. I tried to expect the worse. From my time being a student nurse, every 'oh god' situation I was ever involved in was never good.

I was aware of a rancid smell clouding the air. The first thing I saw was Edward sat upright in his bed, with thick brown vomit all around his mouth, and all up behind him on the wall. Bits of undigested food were everywhere. Thick black particles of undigested food were splattered up the wall behind Edward, and a big pool of dark brown vomit just by his pillow. Edward turned towards me, and spoke a simple 'hello.' Edward spoke in a slow and calm tone with a hint of a Yorkshire accent, oblivious to the vomit around his mouth and up the wall.

As I walked closer up to the bed, I realised that things were going to get a lot worse. Edward was catheter bound. Urinary catheterisation is usually used for people who cannot empty their bladder in the usual way, which could be for a whole manner of reasons. Edward was now far too frail to go to the toilet and lost his mobility a long time ago. It was also helpful to monitor his urine output on a daily basis, and to ensure that everything was draining correctly and efficiently.

Everything was not draining well this morning. Edward was draining blood. And it was everywhere. Emma shouted back to me.

'Go get Paul.'

I rush out onto the corridor and see Paul down the far end.

'Paul! I think we need a hand.'

'What's the problem?'

'It's Edward, he's bleeding everywhere and he's been sick' I blurt out.

'Right okay, I'm on my way.' Paul follows me into Edward's room. Emma had started to clean up around Edward's face with a damp cloth.

Edward was shaking profusely, and had gone a very pale colour.

Paul stood over Edward, and got a small blood sugar monitoring machine out of his tunic.

'Best check his blood sugars whilst were here too.'

Paul got a small lancet needle out, and carefully stated what he was about to do to. Edward nodded in acknowledgement, and Paul gave Edward a very tiny pin prick with the lancet, enough to get a small bubble of blood from his finger, and let it soak into the small strip which was attached to a machine. Once enough blood had dispersed into the strip, it took five seconds to get a reading. We all waited patiently. Edward continued to look up at Paul with his dark brown eyes. The machine beeped.

'Right.'

He showed me the machine.

'1.4mmols'. This was not good. The average range for blood sugar levels should be between 4-7mmols. Anything very low could send someone into a 'hypo' (hypoglycaemic - low blood sugar), or anything very high a hyper (hyperglycaemic – high blood sugar).

Paul threw me the nursing keys and ordered me out of the room.

'Just open up the store cupboard down the hall opposite the sluice mate, and grab us some glucogel, we need to get some sugar into this man quickly.' Emma was continuing to finish cleaning up Edward's mouth.

I rushed out into the hallway and found the store cupboard. I opened it up, my hands were shaking. I inspected the large store cupboard where there were an array of various sizes of needles and cotton wool buds. I scanned quickly for some glucogel. I saw some after what seemed like hours staring into the abyss of the store cupboard, and grabbed it quickly, locked the cupboard, and ran back into Edward's room.

I rushed in to find Paul spoon feeding Edward some weetabix with sugar on top of it, slowly. He quickly put the bowl of weetabix down as he saw me rush in, and I handed him the glucogel.

'Cheers mate.'

Paul ripped open the packet of glucogel and immediately began administering the gel to Edward. Edward looked up at Paul with wonderment.

'Edward, this is just to control your blood sugar levels okay? You need to have this mate.'

Edward remained startled, but he was gradually consuming the glucogel. It took a good five minutes before the bottle was totally drained.

'Right, hopefully that should sort it' Paul shouted out.

'How was that Edward?' he asked.

Edward looked up to Paul and paused for a good ten seconds.

'Right.' He spoke very slowly and surely.

'Have we got anything else to give him?' Paul looked at me.

At university I was always told that you should give someone with low blood sugars a slow release sugary food and a quick release, like a banana and some chocolate.

'What about any bananas?' I ask Paul.

'That might work, have the kitchen got any?' Emma glances to Paul.

'I'll go run down and get some.'

Paul glances down to Edward's penis. It is covered in blood, and the catheter has a very dark and sticky consistency.

'Right, we need a doctor, let's clean him up as best we can, give us a hand will you Jack.'

I follow around to the opposite side of the bed to where Paul is standing. All I can see as I glance down at Edward's groin is a mass of dark sticky blood which has started to infuse itself into the white bed linen. Edward seems oblivious to this blood. Paul starts moving the catheter tube around slowly next to Edward's penis, and small amounts of blood bubble through the tube. My stomach was feeling very queasy; I couldn't quite believe what I was seeing. I glance down again and grab Paul's attention.

'Is that supposed to look like that?' I point down at Edward's penis.

Paul takes a look at the tip of Edward's penis, which appears to be torn.

'Yeh, I'm pretty sure it's always been like that you know'

'Is that...normal?' I enquire.

'Well he is in no pain from it, it's been like that from the day he came here. It doesn't look particularly pleasant though.'

Paul and I gently reposition Edward from side to side, and get him a fresh pair of sheets, and begin cleaning him up. Paul leaves briefly to make a phone call. There was no doctor on call at this home, they would be around a few times in the week, but otherwise it was a call to the local GP practice, or if it was out of hours and the weekend, then there would need to be a phone call made through a special number to doctors that were on call any time.

Edward seemed oblivious to the fuss and commotion he was receiving. As Paul returned he came clutching a handful of chocolate spread sandwiches. He turned to me.

'What about these in the mean time then?'

'Yeah, try it' I say with an air of desperation. Paul begins filling Edward's face. Edward looked up at Paul as he was feeding him. Edward probably felt all his Christmases had come at once. Edward was a big fan of sugar in his earlier years. It was reported that he used to have twenty sugars in his tea and coffee. No wonder he had developed diabetes in his later years. I begin thinking that he must think that he has been awarded the grand prize this morning: Endless sugary food items, coming in at great lengths and speed.

Emma returned clutching a big bowl of mashed up bananas, and put it on Edward's side drawer.

'How we doing then chaps?' Emma shouts out.

'Yeah, err, fine,' I say unconvincingly. Paul turns round, still with a chocolate sandwich in his hand which is halfway down Edward's mouth.

'The doctor's on her way, he may need re-catheterising again' Paul whispers.

Edward had a history of being re-catheterised all too frequently. His catheter would frequently not drain as it should, and often get blocked. A standard catheter should normally last at least three months, but Edward had endured four catheterisations in the past three months alone. I had never seen a catheterisation myself; as mental health nurses we were not trained in any of these general procedures. I had a feeling I would be witness to one this morning, and the thought of it had already made me feel quite light headed.

Paul re-tests Edward's blood sugar levels again. Edward gently raises out a hand in anticipation. Paul gently pricked Edward's finger again, and slowly drew the blood out until the machine had enough blood to start to generate a reading. The next five seconds seemed to last an hour. You could hear a pin drop in this room. Paul looked up at me and wiped his brow.

'2.8. At least were on the right side of things.'

Edward looks towards me with a blank expression on his face. He had barely a few strands of grey hair left and his face was covered with red blisters. He had a wide pronounced nose, and dark brown eyes. His face was quite spherical. He looked like someone you could have a good drink with down the local pub; there was a kind, unthreatening look about him.

'Right, we have cleaned him up at least, I might give him another glucogel just to make sure, and a hot chocolate, and then I will check it again.' Paul rushed off to get another glucogel; I could hear his keys jangling all the way down the corridor. Emma turns to me.

'Right then, I guess we had better crack on getting people up and dressed!'

'Sure thing.'

Paul comes racing back with another glucogel in his hand. Edward turns slowly to him. I begin thinking Edward must be seeing Paul as some kind of sugar fairy, giving him his every wish and command. Paul turns to me and Emma.

'Right, as soon as the doctor's here I'll give you a shout, and I will keep an eye on his blood sugar levels.'

I walk out onto the corridor with Emma.

'Who's next then?'

Edward lets out a very loud cough; he seems to be having trouble clearing his throat. Emma and I looked at each other, and then back at Paul. It was clear we were all thinking the same thing; we were worried that Edward was going to be sick again. Edward watched us all looking at him.

He gradually clears his throat, and immediately closes his eyes and falls back to sleep with his finger pointing up in the air.

We all breathe a sigh of relief. Edward has got a light blue towel wrapped around his neck just in case he is sick.

Emma and I walk out of Edward's room, leaving Paul to finish feeding Edward the last remains of a chocolate sandwich.

As soon as we come out of the corridor I can see Vancy half way down holding on to the wooden handles that are placed all around the walls. She is slowly making her way up the corridor, looking very drained and pale.

'Help.'

'I'm frightened!'

She is making her way very slowly up the corridor and shuffling her feet, looking incredibly unsteady, as she gradually keeps hold of the hand rail.

Emma turns to me.

'Would you mind just trying to settle Vancy down and maybe sit her in the quiet lounge? I'll start on Ella, she just needs a little prompting in room eighty, you can join me in a few minutes'

I start walking towards Vancy. Vancy starts waving at me.

'You sir, yes you, please help me, I say, I say please!'

'Vancy, would you like to come this way please, maybe sit down and come and have a chat with me in the quiet lounge?'

'Well okay then, let's see if we can, but my mother is going to be here any minute, and my father!'

Her parents were obviously not around any more. Long term memory was often still intact with dementia, and frequently people would be able to recall many distant memories including family, but ask them what they had for dinner and they couldn't tell you at all. Sometimes once you spoke a sentence to people they would immediately forget what you had said, moments later.

We slowly walk past the nursing office, where Paul is busily going through the filing cabinets and speaking to someone on the phone at the same time. The office looks chaotic but it is a kind of organised chaos. There are twenty identical red folders on a shelf in the corner which detail each resident's care plans. Below this shelf is another shelf with a few medical books, a stethoscope and an arm cuff, and a box of urine testing strips. The office is very small and cramped but appears to hold everything it needs to.

Just past the nursing office is a smaller lounge known as the quiet lounge; it has a large red plush sofa in it, a few other random chairs, and a fish tank. An old electric organ sits on the far side, opposite the sofa. I steadily walk Vancy into the quiet lounge and sit her on the sofa.

'What's the matter Vancy?' I ask.

'It's no good, I am frightened, frightened I tell you.'

'What are you frightened of?'

'Well I don't know!' Vancy screams.

'I can't help you if I don't know why you are frightened.'

'Well my mother is going to be here soon, and I really need to get her home because she will die otherwise.'

'Vancy, how old are you?'

'Well dear, I don't know, I'm about thirty two I think.'

'Do you know when you were born?'

Vancy pauses for a minute and stares at me.

'I don't know, but I need to get home and find my mother!'

'Vancy you are in your eighties, I don't think your mother and father are around any more.'

'Eighties? No it's not true! It isn't true, you're lying you are, lying I tell you, I must find them.'

'Do you know where you are?'

'I'm not anywhere.'

'Vancy, you are in a private nursing home, this is your home now, you are safe here, this is where you live.'

Vancy's lower lip begins to tremble.

'I am not, you're lying, you are, it's not true, help me, help me, help me, help, help, help, help, help, help, help, please!'

Vancy was actually shaking quite rapidly and frothing at the mouth a little. Her hands were raised a little and she started to edge herself off the sofa very slowly.

Telling the truth with people with dementia was one of the hardest judgements to make. You could either go along with their perceived reality, or you could tell them the truth and try to orientate them to time and place. Sometimes neither would work, and sometimes you would pick the wrong option; sometimes you simply had to use your own sixth sense and just go with it. It was massively difficult and something you couldn't always learn in a lecture theatre.

Vancy was continuing to edge herself more and more off the sofa.

'Help me will you, I must find my mother.'

'Vancy, would you like anything to drink?'

'No, I must get off now, I'm afraid.'

I gradually help Vancy stand up off the sofa, before she falls off it. Vancy starts walking towards the door and off out into the corridor. Wandering was also common of dementia and one that couldn't really be solved. We can either medicate people until they have no will or strength left in them to walk, or we can try to minimise the risk, by having as safe an environment as possible. It is impossible to completely eliminate any form of risk, but we can certainly minimise it. Wandering behaviour could be for a whole manner of things; Vancy was clearly in distress and trying to find her mother. Sometimes people will think of something they want to do and forget half way through walking and get confused and disorientated.

Vancy needed to be allowed the freedom and choice to walk around the unit, despite her being at a risk of falling. Unfortunately what would usually happen is people would eventually fall so much or so badly that they could end up having a very serious injury and eventually become bed bound.

It made me really nervous when people who were at high risk of falls were walking around hospitals; I always panicked about the possibility of them falling and what I could do to help them. Initial instinct is often to try and break their fall, but I was always told not to as it could cause more damage to either the patient or yourself. I had tried to calm down Vancy as much as I could, but if people want to leave, they will, and if people want to walk, they will. We cannot restrain or obstruct someone's free will, regardless of risk.

I walk out of the quiet lounge and watch Vancy walk up the corridor. Paul had come out of the nursing office and was clutching a small plastic medicine pot with a plastic spoon in it.

'I think I had better give her some Lorazepam don't you?'

'Yeh, I think it might be needed,' I say.

Paul goes marching up the corridor after Vancy, who has picked up quite a pace now in her walking speed. Paul comes round to the front of her.

'Vancy, I just have a tablet for you.'

'Help, help, no I'm frightened.'

I follow up the corridor, just behind Vancy.

Paul tries again, and gently eases the plastic spoon into Vancy's mouth; Vancy automatically opens her mouth and takes the small tablet. She immediately pulls a face and starts trying to remove the tablet out of her mouth with her hand.

'No I don't want this, it tastes horrible.'

Paul gently takes her hand and pops the tablet back into the medicine pot, and tries again.

Vancy won't even take the spoon near her mouth now; she is off on her own mission. Paul walks past me with a deep sigh. Vancy carries on walking right up to the end of the unit next to the exit door. She is looking out of the small window pane to the door.

'Help me, help me, help me, help me, help me, help me, help me, helllllllpppp.'

Paul turns to me.

'Well, that didn't go down too well, I might have to try again later when she has calmed down a little, this is the usual pattern sometimes, she might settle and sleep after lunchtime hopefully.'

Paul walks back towards the nursing office. I go to find Emma in room eighty.

Sharon and Katie were coming out of the various rooms, dropping off the dirty laundry into the laundry trolleys situated in the corridor. There were two laundry trolleys, one each side of the unit, colour coded for convenience. Red for infected or soiled linen, white for standard linen, and blue for patient's clothes. The standard procedure after getting someone up, washed and dressed was to strip the bed of all the sheets, and replace them with fresh ones, open the curtains and windows, and generally make sure the room was tidy and presentable.

I would never be able to master the art of hospital corners I thought to myself, but I tried to not let that bother me this morning. At university we had a whole session on how to make the beds. I was often laughed at for my appalling bed making skills, I had to hang my head in shame and claim that I was merely a 'bloke', whilst really thinking that I was sure it didn't matter that much, there must be more important things I needed to learn whilst I was there, and this morning I had bigger problems to deal with.

Suddenly an alarm bell rang. It was a very shrill sound, and rang twice, and repeated, not like a telephone ring, but more an abrupt short snappy ring. There were boxes on the wall that alerted the staff to what room it was being rung in. Every room had a large red piece of string attached to a buzzer. Some of the patients who had more capacity could use these bells to help alert staff to any needs they had.

'Who's that?' I say to Sharon.

'Don't worry baby, that's probably just Elsie, room sixty five. She is quite anxious, panics about being got up. Go and see her and tell her we will be there in a minute.' I walk down the other end of the corridor and into room sixty five.

There is a lady sat up in her bed in a pink dressing gown. She has a table that is over her bed, with two empty yoghurt pots on it and a fresh cup of tea.

Elsie would frequently ring the bell a number of times in a morning, sometimes even before handover. This used to rile the carers and it got on their nerves. It seemed no matter how much persuasion you gave Elsie that she would be getting up, a few moments later she would still ring the bell. I think she had a misconception about how much time had passed, and a few moments to her might feel like many more minutes. You could guarantee if the bell was ringing it would be Elsie who was wanting to get up and go to the lounge area.

Elsie had two supportive daughters who used to visit her often, and some weekends would take Elsie home for a couple of nights. Elsie didn't always appear to enjoy this trip away, but other times she would look forward to it. It was nice that Elsie still had the opportunity for a change of scenery, but the daughters would frequently feel the burden of looking after their mother for a weekend. It was getting more and more difficult to mobilise Elsie, and often she would complain of being bored, but the daughters carried on as best they could.

One of the daughters was a doctor, the other a clinical psychologist, so they were very on the ball when it came to their mother's medication, and would often suggest different doses or new medications to the nurses, who would then pass this information on to the doctor. Sometimes being so close to the same field could be a hindrance. A lot of the nurses felt that way sometimes, but at the end of the day, everyone was here to try and do their best for Elsie.

I walk into Elsie's room and introduce myself.

'Hello, I'm Jack, how can I help you?'

'Who are you?' Elsie asks.

Elsie has permed white hair and bright green eyes, with a squarish face.

'I'm Jack; I'm a nurse who's just started to work here!'

'Is someone going to get me up?'

'Yes, they're just getting people up now, so they won't be long.'

'Who's going to get me up? Is Sharon on?'

'Yes, Sharon's on, and Paul'

'Is Paul doing the tablets?'

'Yes Paul is doing the tablets, he won't be long either.'

'I don't want to be here all day, is someone going to be getting me up soon then? I get frightened that I will be left here all day.'

'You won't be here all day; they won't be long at all, I promise.'

I step outside the room and follow round to where Paul is sitting in the office. Jennifer suddenly comes barging through the other door which is connected to the main lounge, from another unit. She is clutching large amounts of paper in her hand and walking speedily towards me and Paul.

'How many staff have you got on today?'

Paul glances up at the rota which is stuck firmly on the wall with bright pink 'blu' tack.

'Now then let's see, five in the morning, five in the afternoon.'

'Nope, you won't do then, I'll have to try and rob someone from downstairs.'

A daily check on the rota by Jennifer would normally happen each morning. Frequently it might be needed to swap the odd carer around to some of the other units, if other units were short in staffing numbers. This would anger the carers, as they could be swapped to a unit they were not familiar with. It was in your contract that you could be required to work in any area if needed, and night shifts too. A lot of the carers would simply refuse to do nights, and threaten to leave the company if they were given any.

Jennifer turns to me.

'I'll need you to sign an induction form too and your contract. How are you getting on with the chaos so far?'

'Oh fine,' I say.

'Wait till you're properly in charge, that's when the fun begins!' She walks off equally as fast as she came in.

There should always be one qualified nurse on, and four carers on this unit. Some carers and nurses did 8 a.m. – 2 p.m. shifts, and some would do 2 p.m. – 8 p.m. shifts. As long as the balance always worked out to five staff members all day, everyone was happy. This was very rarely the case though. Staff members would get robbed, pinched, swapped and moved around consistently to try and balance all the units' staffing needs. This meant potential strain on the unit if you were running understaffed.

This unit was the heaviest out of the entire home, so the staffing levels were vital. To keep everything running smoothly and efficiently you needed to be running with five staff each and every day. On rare occasions you would get six staff in the morning and five in the afternoon, and ultra rarely six staff members all day long. A happy team was a productive team. It had started to get worse here; morale was at an all time low.

Staffing levels

'Short staffing compromises care both directly and indirectly. Recurrent short staffing results in increased staff stress and reduced staff wellbeing, leading to higher sickness absence (needing more bank and agency cover), and more staff leaving.'

Royal College of Nursing, (2010)

In the home, five people left in one month, and they attributed their main reasons for leaving as short staffing the unit too regularly, not feeling safe, and not feeling like they had enough time to spend with the residents as they were continually involved in 'task based' activities.

In a single month the home had spent over £3,500 on agency staff. Agency staff often cost more than regular staff; an agency carer will cost the company £9.49 an hour on weekdays, compared to a regular member of staff costing around £6 an hour. £11.91 on week nights and Saturday, £14.89 on Sunday and £19.65 per hour on a bank holiday. Under no circumstances would the home ever employ an agency nurse, they wouldn't ever contemplate it; they beg, borrow and steal staff as much as they can. If this meant the manager had to come in and cover a shift, then she would, rather than pay for the additional rates that a nurse would cost.

'In care homes there is an average ratio of 18 patients per registered nurse during the day, and 26 patients at night.'

Nurses can often feel:

- Stretched to the limits
- Report that they have insufficient time to deliver care properly
- Have higher levels of stress
- Are not refreshed and rested (often skipping breaks and working overtime to fill staffing gaps)

'In hospital wards, an average of 5.4 nursing staff are on duty during the daytime – roughly three registered nurses and two HCA's / auxiliaries per ward.'

Nursing Homes regulation and Quality Improvement Authority, (2009)

The home would normally aim to operate with one registered nurse with three to four care assistants. Sometimes there would be two registered nurses, with either two to three care assistants.

Whenever I was the only nurse in charge, with only three care assistants, I would frequently have difficulty grabbing a break. It would often be 3 p.m. before I even got off the ward. Being the only nurse in charge meant that everyone always wanted to speak to you. If there was a doctor's round in the morning, then it would be near impossible to grab your morning break. You were stuck in every direction; everyone wanted a piece of you. Relatives would ring constantly in the morning, often during the medication round.

You would also be speaking to relatives in person, documenting changes, dealing with any falls or dressings. The workload was intense and constant. At times you really had to fight to get off the ward and relax. Many a time I have been called back from the staff room because a resident has fallen over, cutting my break short. Operating on pure adrenalin at times is not healthy in the long run, running on constant levels of stress.

The following are offered as guideline for staff : patient ratios;

'Propose nursing homes staffed so that over 24-hour period there is an average of 35 percent registered nurses and 65 percent care assistants.'

- Early shifts – 1:5
- Late shifts – 1:6
- Night – 1:10

Royal College of Nursing, (2010)

The home would often try to aim for one member of staff for every five residents. One nurse and three care assistants would meet this recommendation; however it does not take into account the skill mix, or the resident mix.

The more residents that are aggressive, mobile, and prone to falls will increase the risk, and require more intervention. Staff at the home would always feel safer with at least one nurse and four care assistants on every shift.

With two nurses and three care assistants, then the second nurse worked as a carer for the duration of the shift, but was also on hand to offer nursing interventions and complete documentation, but their primary role is that of a carer.

Extracts taken from Royal College of Nursing: Guidance on safe nurse staffing levels in the UK, (2010)

'The research evidence demonstrates that there is an association between nurse staffing and patient outcomes. There is no universal truth about the number of nurses needed, and no short cuts to identifying the optimal level. Services and the staff required to provide them must be shaped on the basis of patient need.'

From: RCN Policy position: evidence – based nurse staffing levels, (2010)

There was an instance, on a night shift where the night nurse had to be in charge of both units, with only two agency carers on the one unit, leaving her upstairs to look after twenty residents personal care needs. She was furious, and that morning many residen'ts bed sheets had to be changed as they were soaking in urine. She simply hadn't got all the resources she needed to give everyone the time that they needed. She put in a complaint with the management, and the owner swiftly replied back saying that she was sorry that the staffing levels were at 'bare bones' that night, but she still stated that this was perfectly legal. Forty residents were being managed by 3 members of staff, 2 agency carers, and one mental health nurse, over two floors.

> 'More than 75% of nurses fear for their patients' safety because of inadequate staffing levels, poor ward layout and the bad attitude of colleagues'
>
> **Nursing Times, (2011)**

The night shifts worked a little differently. There would be one nurse and one carer to run an entire shift. Sometimes a nurse would have to run two units. Paul told me horror stories about some of the night nurses who had to run two units, being responsible for up to forty residents on their own, with two carers per unit.

All of the nurses felt uncomfortable working two units; they felt that it was a lot riskier. The other unit was downstairs, and anything could happen on a night shift. There would be two carers working on each unit, and the nurse would split their time between both units, depending on where they were needed. This also meant that they would have to do both sets of nursing notes.

The main problem the nurses had was the extra element of risk. What if there was a death on one of the units? What if two incidents happened, one on each unit? What if two people fell, and the nurse had to sort both incidents out, on different units? They were doubling the element of risk.

When the nurses tried to contest this, they were often told by the management that they had 'every faith in them' and shrugged their concerns off, and the nurses dutifully carried on despite voicing their concerns. Another nurse threatened not to work two units, and said that she wouldn't accept the keys, if she was going to be forced into working with double the amount of residents. She put her concerns in writing, and was told that if she didn't like it, then she could look for another job. She was told that from time to time it had to be accepted that a nurse would be required to work both units.

Another nurse took it one step further and wrote an email to the NMC. They replied, saying that they don't provide standards or publish guidance on staffing levels, as it remains a workforce issue.

NMC Environment of Care

'Nurses and midwives are often faced with concerns regarding the environment of care where the interest and safety of people in their care are at risk. They face a dilemma of how to remedy this. Nurses and midwives who are concerned that a situation may obstruct the achievement of satisfactory standards may then risk censure from their employers. On the other hand, failure to make concerns known renders nurses and midwives vulnerable to a complaint to the NMC for failing to satisfy standards of public protection. This may place their registration status in jeopardy. The code makes clear what is expected of them. This is a vital tool in delivering effective public protection'. The code states that nurses and midwives must:

'Work with others to protect and promote the health and wellbeing of those in your care, their families and carers, and the wider community"

> They are also required to 'manage risk'. The responsibilities of nurses and midwives are that they:
>
> "Must act without delay if you believe that you, a colleague or anyone else may be putting someone at risk."
>
> "Must inform someone in authority if you experience problems that prevent you working within this code or other nationally agreed standards."
>
> "Must report your concerns in writing if problems in the environment of care are putting people at risk."
>
> 'An essential part in the reporting process is the making of contemporaneous and accurate records demonstrating the potential shortfalls in the care required by people in the care of nurses and midwives. If complaints are made about nurses and midwives involved in delivering care, managers should be able to confirm that the perceived inadequacies in the environment of care had been drawn to their attention and that records to this effect have been maintained.'
> **(NMC, 2008)**

The nurses were understandably worried about the safety element, and their registration and fitness to practice, if anything was to go wrong on a night shift, and they ultimately took full responsibility for this.

I walk back up the corridor to join Emma. Emma is already walking out of a room towards me.

'Ella is fine, she just needed a little help with her jumper, we need to do Dwayne next.'

'Okay.'

'And we will need the hoist.'

I remember the hoist from my student days, another piece of equipment that would help you move a resident from their chair or bed and transport them to a wheelchair or back to bed. It reminded me of a mini crane or JCB, as it had all sorts of fancy controls on it whereby you could tilt the resident and move them up and down. They sat in a cloth sling, and were perfectly safe in it. During our student classes we all had the chance to experience what it was like sitting in a sling and being transported around. The experience was scary as you didn't feel particularly safe, so I always wondered what it must feel like for someone who has dementia and is already very confused.

I drag the hoist out from the bathroom and follow Emma towards Dwayne's room. I can still hear Dwayne shouting away to himself as I walk into the room with the hoist and Emma.

'No no no no no nonononononono Johnny!'

Dwayne is very agitated, and he is staring right at me, and shaking his fists.

Emma tries to calm him down.

'Dwayne, were just going to be a few minutes and get you up washed and dressed.'

Dwayne looks up at Emma and stops shouting for a brief second.

'Alright then.'

'Right, we need pants, socks, and the rest,' Emma commands me.

If residents had the capacity to make a choice then it was always good practice to give them a choice in what they wished to wear. Dwayne did not have this capacity. I grab some pants and socks for him, and pick out a vest and a shirt and trousers, and place them on the side of the chair by the bed.

Emma had gone into the bathroom and was preparing a small bowl of hot soapy water, gathering her flannel, towel, wipes, and deodorant.

She walked back into the room with all her equipment, and placed it on a table right beside the bed. Dwayne was sat bolt upright.

'Dwayne, we are just going to take your vest off.'

Dwayne doesn't respond. Emma and I gradually start taking Dwayne's vest off. He is very rigid, not assisting in any way. I can already begin to feel myself sweat as we gradually ease his vest off.

'Now just watch his hands whilst I give him a wash.'

Many a time I have had to carefully keep a resident's hands close to mine in case of any sudden jolts and hitting out, always aware of personal space.

Dwayne appeared quite relaxed as Emma was washing him; his hands were moving a little. Once Emma had finished washing his top half, and dried it, we started to gradually put his clothes on. After putting on his vest, we then started to put his shirt on. There is nothing more strenuous and energy zapping than trying to put on a resident's clothing who is actively trying to resist.

Dwayne's arms were flailing about, and his shirt was going everywhere. I tried to hold his hands whilst Emma desperately tried to find his arm to put through the arm of his shirt.

'No no no no leave it leave it leave it leave it leave it will you!'

I could feel a few beads of sweat forming on my nose, and my back beginning to ache a fraction. Emma eventually got the one arm in, and then passed the shirt around Dwayne's back for me to put his other arm through. My arm got a little close to Dwayne's mouth, and Dwayne started to try and bite my arm. Eventually, after much tugging and stretching of fabric, Dwayne had got his shirt on.

Doing up shirt buttons with latex gloves on had to rank as one of the hardest tasks to do quickly and efficiently. I could feel Dwayne's hot breath, breathing down on me as I was doing up his buttons. I took a few attempts at each button, and the more he writhed about, the harder I found it to do the buttons up. Eventually I managed it, and Emma helped me to roll Dwayne over onto his right hand side, so he was facing me. Emma took off his incontinence pad, and began cleaning his lower half.

Dwayne was trying to grab my tunic and I was desperately trying to avoid him doing this, whilst also holding him still so that Emma could clean him. Emma moves a pillow slowly around under Dwayne's head to make him a little more comfortable. She turns her nose up and rolls her eyes.

'Oh, that's just disgusting.' Emma stares at the pillow.

The pillow has a pillowcase over it, but there is a resident's name clearly inscribed on the pillow underneath the case.

'She died over eight months ago! That's absolutely disgusting, how can you re use pillows like that! That is a total MRSA risk, imagine the dead skin cells, and bodily fluids, and dandruff, all contained in there. God, this place gets me down!'

Emma finishes cleaning Dwayne. She had got a bright green pad ready. It was a tag pad, similar to a baby's nappy, but had two small sticky tags that would wrap around the hips and stick the pad into position each side. The tag pads held a lot more than some of the other pads, and could hold up to four litres of urine at any one time.

There were all different sorts of pads which were assessed for use with each resident depending on their incontinence needs. The pad list would cause no end of gripes and complaints with everyone. Everyone was assigned a particular amount of pads for the working day. The home would strictly stand by this list, as, depending on whether the residents were self funding or not, meant that they would only be allocated a certain amount of pads for each day.

It would be very difficult to say exactly how incontinent a dementia patient was throughout a typical day. This would cause rifts between management and staff; it was totally dependent on the day and the resident. Some of the carers had even resorted to locking some of the pads away so that they couldn't be returned by the maintenance man and the unit would have plenty of spare pads if they needed them. I heard that one day the whole home ran out of pads due to an ordering error. The same day a severe outbreak of diarrhoea and vomiting occurred. The maintenance man had to make a hasty trip to go and get some more.

As long as you were always acting in the best interests of the resident, no one could say anything against you. If someone needed an additional pad, then they would get one. What would be the alternative? Ringing the manager to state that 'Mrs X' had run out of her allotted pads for the day, so she wouldn't be getting any more? It just wouldn't happen.

We needed to get Dwayne's trousers on, which we did very efficiently as Dwayne had seemed to calm down more now. Emma started getting the sling ready for Dwayne, and with a few rolls and repositions. Dwayne was fully clipped into the sling, ready to be attached to the hoist. We manoeuvre him deftly into his wheelchair, and I start to wheel him into the lounge area, with Emma following behind me making a lot of clattering noises as the hoist rolls over the carpet in the corridor.

Once in the lounge area, we re-attach Dwayne to the hoist. He is starting to shout a little again and I narrowly miss him trying to hit my groin area. We slowly move him into his chair, and put his feet up a little in the recliner.

'Right, can you just put the hoist back in Mark's room please? We won't need this for now.'

'Sure.'

Emma didn't look fazed. She had been doing the job a while, and she knew what she was doing. I slowly tear off my blue apron, still feeling the sweat pouring from me. I enter the sluice room and take off my gloves and wash my hands.

The sluice room was a very tiny room with two sinks in it, and three mops and buckets crammed in it, with a couple of clinical waste bins opposite the sinks. The carers would be in and out of this room after dealing with each and every patient. The sounds of the clinical waste bin creaking up and down would be continual throughout the morning as the carers threw each bag of waste from each of the resident's rooms.

As I exit the sluice room, it slams shut behind me. Emma joins me outside. She thrusts me another blue plastic apron.

'Right, just one bath to do now, then we are done. Our friend Fred.'

There was a bath list for everybody. Most residents would get bathed once a week, on set days. If they were too frail then they would often get a bed bath instead. The residents would be offered a choice of a shower or bath sometimes. If the unit was feeling the pressure due to a shortage of staff, residents would often get showered rather than a 'time consuming' bath, and sometimes just a quick bed bath. These were often the areas that got missed. Sharon would often tell residents that they were having a shower on bath day, to save time for the unit, rather than give them a choice. Unfortunately these were just some of the areas that would get omitted during days of lower staff levels. It was the residents that ultimately would miss out.

'If you can start running the bath, I will go get Fred and his clothes for him, he has some bath stuff in there already with his name on it.'

I enter the bathroom. Luckily it is very similar to the ones I used during my student nurse training. A couple of press buttons, and a keypad in order to operate the bath chair electronically, to move it up and out of the bath, in order to get your resident safely in.

I begin running the water and spot Fred's bubble bath on the side. I turn the bottle upside down ready to give it a quick press. The cap comes flying off and a huge glob of bubble bath splashes into the water. I hastily retrieve the bubble bath cap and put the bottle back on the side. The bath is already starting to fill a little more deeply with light foam.

Emma comes bursting through the bathroom door with an armful of clothes and towels.

'Right, I think that's everything, we just need Fred now! He's lovely, originally from London, he has great comprehension, and you can have a laugh and a joke with him.'

'Excellent,' I say. I am trying to guard the rising foam from behind me in the bath. I swirl the water round and check the temperature. There is a good four feet of foam now piled high in the bath. Soft fluffy bath foam clouds float around the bathroom.

Emma comes back wheeling in a small old gentleman with thick gold frame glasses. He waves his hand up in the air.

'Hello sir!'

By now I cannot hide the fact that the bathroom is filled with foam.

'Jesus Jack what did you do!' Emma shouts out.

Fred is smiling from ear to ear.

'Cor blimey son, this is a real bubble bath today then!'

Emma and I begin undressing Fred, and sit him onto the white bath hoist chair, gently lifting him up in the chair, through the thick blanket of foam. Fred is kicking some of the foam bubbles that are floating past him. He finally gets lowered into the bath.

'Oh I say this is a turn up for the books.'

'Well Fred, this is like a spa treatment this morning!'

We all start bursting out into laughter. I have never seen so much foam in one bathroom in all my life. It is so hot I can feel my top damp with sweat already. Fred looks in his element. A big layer of foam is stuck to his glasses.

'I can hardly see here my old mate.'

I quickly wipe the foam off Fred's glasses. Emma starts to wash his hair; she cannot stop herself from laughing hard.

Fred is also laughing along with us. He is kicking and swatting the foam clouds as they come past. Fred even laughs and chuckles in a very cockney sounding way.

'I certainly will be clean for me mam today that's for sure.'

'We will have to charge you extra for this Fred! Bubbles come as an additional extra don't you know!'

'Well, okay, just put it on my tab and we can settle up later.'

We all burst out laughing again and look at the absurdity of the situation. We eventually manage to clean Fred up, remove most of the foam off him, and give him a good drying off.

Emma wheels Fred out to the lounge area. As I walk past to pop the towels in the laundry I see Paul coming out of the nursing office. Fred shouts out to Paul.

'Hello sir, now I wanted to ask you something.'

'Fire away my mate!' Paul answers.

'Now you know these tablets I am on. How long do I have to be on them for?'

'Well Fred, for the meantime at least a good few months.'

'Right, I thought so, and these will keep me level will they, keep me on the straight and narrow?'

'They sure will.'

'Okay, I just wanted to know that's all. I don't mind taking them, some people they don't bother do they, they just spit them out or throw 'em on the floor. I always think how are you ever going to get better if you don't take your tablets?'

Fred lifts both his arms up and gives a big shrug. He smiles at Paul.

'Some people just don't care do they, they don't realise that the medication can help you.'

'They sure don't Fred. If only everyone could be like you, then we wouldn't have any problems at all.'

Fred laughs out loud.

'Simple to me, you're the boss, I will keep taking them then and listen to any new orders from you boss. I feel fine anyway; look, I can move my legs up and down now.'

Fred moves his legs up and down.

'Excellent' Paul replies.

'Simple. Just keep taking the tablets I say, and keep going.'

'Words to live by Fred. Words to live by.'

'Listen now, do you think there is going to be any way that I can go home today? I really want to go home but I doubt they will let me today.'

'Not today I'm afraid, Fred.'

Fred looks down into his open palmed hands, looking a little sad.

'Well, at the end of the day, they make the rules, and we pay the money I guess.'

Emma wheels Fred into the lounge area. I follow behind her, a few moments later and Paul shouts to me.

'The doctor's here to look at Edward. Come with me, I'm going to need your help.'

10–11 a.m.

Paul and I walk into Edward's room. There is a young female doctor with a large briefcase, which is open, containing a number of plastic tubes and needles in a big pile.

'Hi, I'm Dr. Litten. When was he last catheterised?'

Paul thinks for a few moments.

'I think it was only a few weeks ago; I can double check, but it wasn't long ago.'

Dr. Litten nods.

'I think I am going to have to change it anyway, looking at this.'

She walks over to Edward, touches his penis lightly and a small pool of blood seeps out. My stomach does a double flip, I try to hide my nausea.

Dr. Litten begins unpacking various tubes and an assortment of cloths. Paul goes around to the side of Edward's bed and directs me to the opposite side. Dr Litten brings out a small clear tube of something, and gradually places it on the tip of Edward's penis.

'This will help numb the pain Edward.'

She squeezes what appears to be a gel directly into the opening of his urethra, and Edward groans a little.

Dr. Litten gently pulls on the tube to Edward's catheter and slowly draws it out. Edward groans again as the tube slowly comes out; small clumps of blood can be seen on the tube, a dirty dark brown colour.

Dr. Litten removes the old tube and quickly re-inserts a brand new tube. Edward groans a little, but the procedure is done remarkably quickly, and the catheter bag instantly starts to drain with thick dark brown/red murky fluid.

'It's going to look quite dark for a day or so, but keep pushing with fluids and that should clear up soon, and let's just go from there.'

Dr. Litten begins packing up her briefcase again, and passes me the old catheter tube and bag which is still stuck together with congealed blood. I quickly pop it in a clear plastic bag, ready to be disposed of in the clinical waste bin.

Dr. Litten thanks both of us for our help, and walks out of the door and out of the unit.

Paul looks at me.

'Well, that's that then, bet you're glad you came today aren't you mate!'

Paul smiles at me, and I smile back. Edward has gone immediately back to sleep, seemingly oblivious as to what has just gone on. We tidy up the room a little, and leave Edward to rest.

Around 10:30 a.m. the morning drinks need to be prepared. This will often be a choice of squash, blackcurrant or orange. I get an assortment of clear plastic jugs and place them onto the grey trolley, and begin wheeling the trolley into the lounge area. The lounge is still quiet, but it now contains at least eight or nine residents.

I begin filling up the large jugs with squash. The squash is contained in industrial sized five litre plastic bottles. The squash is the cheapest you can buy, sugar free and complete with as many E numbers as you could think of, and Aspartame sweetener. It is such a shame that the elderly residents are often given the cheapest products going. In their minds, I guess people think that it is okay. I don't; these are supposed to be the 'golden years'. There isn't much golden about the quality choices on offer here. I arrange the plastic beakers and mugs on the trolley and pour out the drinks, making a mixture of both orange and blackcurrant.

A lot of the carers find making the morning drinks a real chore. Some have come up with ingenious ways to let others do the drinks. Often the carers slow themselves down a little when they are coming to the end of getting residents up. Some pretend to still be washing or dressing a resident, when really they are just sitting in the residents' room watching television, hoping that the other carers will have finished their side, and then have to start the drinks.

The carers often finish so that they won't have to start doing the morning drinks, and then go off for their break, so that by the time they get back all the drinks will have been completed. Often, they try and get the nurse to do the morning drinks for them, saying that they simply are not going to have enough time. It had started to become an expectation of all the carers that this job would be done either by the nurse, or other carers that could be manipulated into it. They appear to continually come up with new tweaks to the system, in order to allow themselves as many breaks as possible. They have a plan as to how they want their day to go. Carefully constructed smoking breaks certainly appear a big part of it.

By this time of the day, the cleaners will be out in force. I have spotted one of them already, a tiny Polish lady by the name of Ilandria. All the cleaners wear bright purple polo shirts, and often go undetected on the unit, cleaning each resident's room slowly but surely. Most of the cleaners are on minimum wage, a few pence over six pounds an hour, and just 12p an hour extra for working weekends.

Ilandria has been under particular scrutiny by the rest of the cleaning team. They don't like how she does her job. Ilandria is about 5 feet 2 inches, with short greasy blonde hair, and thick brown framed glasses. She rarely speaks to you, except to say the odd greeting in the morning if you are lucky.

Ilandria has been getting a lot of complaints lately from most of the other cleaners and laundry staff. Most people want Ilandria to be sacked. But she can't be; she owes the company thousands of pounds.

Ilandria clocks in to work each morning around 9 a.m., and by about 9:30 a.m. she will be out in the smoking shelter, having her first cigarette break of the day. She then saunters back onto the unit, does some hoovering, and cleans a resident's room. After each room she has cleaned, she can often be spotted again in the smoking shelter having a break. The cleaners are entitled to the same amount of breaks as everyone else, a maximum of three throughout the working day. According to some reports, Ilandria can have up to ten breaks on any given day. If approached about this, Ilandria will complain and say that she is being victimised because of her nationality, so everyone tends to back off. A year ago, she started getting behind with her rent, and needed new ways to pay for her monthly bills. She approached the home with her predicament, and the home dutifully loaned her a thousand pounds, to be paid back over the course of the next few months, directly out of her wages. This worked well for a while, until Ilandria, become more and more indebted to the company, and had to ask for more and more money as the months went on.

The cleaning staff began to notice that a lot of their cleaning supplies were being diminished rather too quickly. They suspected Ilandria as the chief culprit, and along with a detailed search of everyone's locker, they demanded Ilandria to open hers. She wouldn't, so the management opened the locker anyway. What they found was at least a month's supply of cleaning materials stashed in her locker. When quizzed about this, Ilandria said that she had no money to afford to buy cleaning products for her home.

The management pondered the situation for a while, and gave Ilandria a warning; they declined to sack her as she still owed them a considerable amount of money. They decided to brush the matter under the carpet, keeping Ilandria on working and paying her debt off. The cleaning and laundry staff continue to complain about her working practice.

The laundry girls collect the previous night's laundry out of the trolleys and anything that was already filled up from the morning's activities. They are pleasant ladies and always seem to be working hard. They will soon be here, bustling away, getting out the huge sacks of laundry from the previous night's shift. The whole unit runs on team work; everyone has his or her role, and without any particular cog in the machine, everything would collapse.

There is also a team of Thai ladies, recently employed in the cleaning department, for their hard working attitude. They wanted to work every single day of the week, to send money back home to their families, they just couldn't understand English working time directives, no matter how many times it was explained to them. They were driving the rest of the cleaners mad. They would often argue with each other, bicker outside the manager's office, and accuse the other cleaners of being rude to them, racist, and ignoring them. They would keep their own interesting food items piled high in the fridge, a concoction of fish, vegetables and noodles, all stored in individual plastic containers, enough to feed an entire family each, much to the annoyance of the other cleaners and laundry staff.

Paul is in the office starting his handover template on the computer. He often starts early, and gets some of the basic details of each resident and then adds to it during the day, so he has a comprehensive and detailed handover by the end of the day for the night staff.

The phone rings sharply. Paul answers it. He comes rushing down the corridor to me.

'Jack, sorry mate, I need a quick favour from you; Green Unit desperately needs a male carer to shower a gentleman they have who is refusing to be showered by any of the female carers. Do you mind just going down there and quickly showering him? It's just a quick shower and dress, shouldn't take more than about ten minutes tops.'

I was immediately hit by a sense of panic. I tried not to show it to Paul.

'Sure thing, where do I go?'

'It's just the unit downstairs, straight down the stairs, past reception, follow the signs around. They are going to send someone up in your place whilst you're away, that's the deal, so just make sure they do that before you start.'

'Okay.'

'I'm sorry to do this to you; this unit gets all the bad breaks, they're always after us for something! It won't take long at all though, you will be back here in no time, don't worry.'

I make my way around, down the stairs to Green unit, an exact replica of the unit I had just come from. I follow round to the nursing station. There are a few staff members in the office. I introduce myself, and an incredibly tall nurse comes to my aid. She must be at least six and a half foot.

'Hi, thanks for coming down, the gentleman is just down the corridor, I'll show you to him. He's quite new to us, he came in with his wife just a few days ago. Just see how you get on. The wife will just stay in the room. She will be fine, just press the alarm bell if you need anything.'

I enter into the room, immediately surprised at the amount of clutter in the room. There are pants and socks everywhere, pictures strewn all over the wall in a seemingly nonsensical order. Matthew was sat, huddled in the corner of the room, just finishing off his breakfast; he was dressed in the top half of his pyjamas, and a small pair of white briefs.

'Hello, my name's Jack, I'm just here to help you to get up washed and dressed.'

Matthew turns to me slowly. He has wispy greying hair and a posh manner to his voice.

'No that's quite all right really, I will be fine.'

'It's okay, I'm a nurse, I just need to give you a quick shower.'

'Oh no, it's quite all right, I don't need a shower, it's fine, honestly.'

I start to prepare Matthew's clothes for him. I spot his wardrobe, and begin taking a few choice items of clothing out, getting all the necessary items ready. I show Matthew a couple of his shirts and ask him which he would prefer.

'Oh, it's quite all right, I'll pick that one kind sir, the blue one with stripes.'

I gradually collect his clothes together.

Matthew is still drinking his tea, but is pulling a face at it.

'I say, have you got any boiling water, this tea has gone cold you know.'

'I will get you some after your shower Matthew, don't worry.'

Matthews's wife was still lying in bed, a little upright; she was watching my every move.

'I say dear, can you tell me why I am here, where am I?'

'You're in a nursing home.'

'And how long have I been here?'

'Only a few days.'

'Why have I been placed here? You see my husband and I are very confused as to what we are doing here, so if you could shed any light on the matter I would be more than grateful.'

There was an immense pressure to place residents within the home; beds meant money. Assessments would often be done quickly, usually by

Jennifer (an RGN) and beds would be filled almost immediately, however not necessarily for the greater good of the resident involved. When people did appear to be inappropriately placed, the staffing level still appeared weak.

In the past, the owner has promised friends of hers that their relatives can have a room at the home, despite the residents being settled in an existing nursing home. Nurses are frequently heard to say 'I thought this was a nursing home, for frail, elderly people with end stage dementia, not an assessment ward where you have to drug people, and have them sectioned because they're not appropriately placed or assessed!' There had been a few instances where residents had been offered a place at the home without any formal assessment.

The home was traditionally a no smoking home for all residents; however, one of the residents was allowed to smoke whenever he chose to. Out of all eighty residents, one resident was allowed this luxury. His son was very good friends with the owner.

'Sure thing, I will get another nurse to come and speak to you afterwards, I'm just going to give Matthew a shower and get him dressed.'

'Okay love, you carry on, although I'm bursting for the toilet, can I just use it first?'

'Of course, you have plenty of time.'

Matthew's wife slowly moves up out of her bed and walks slowly towards the en suite toilet in the room in a vivid green dressing gown.

Matthew was still staring long and hard into his cup of tea.

'There's still no damn boiling water you know, can you get me some please?'

'After I have given you a wash, no problem.'

Matthews wife comes out a short while later, and casts me a short glance.

'Right, that's a lot better, I was bursting, I'm feeling a little dizzy actually, I'll just go back to bed I think. You will find out why we're here won't you ? It has been most confusing for both of us you know.'

'I will, don't worry.'

'Matthew, come with me please, I will take you to the bathroom and get you a shower.'

'I don't want a shower my good man, I already told you that.'

'Okay, a quick wash and dress then.'

I gradually encourage Matthew to follow me. He seems keen on getting his clothes on, so I gradually manage to walk him into his bathroom. Matthew puts his pants on straight away, whilst I turn my back.

'Matthew, can I just give you a quick shower please?'

'No I told you enough times already sir, I have a shower in the evening.'

I decide to stop asking Matthew for a shower; it was clear he wasn't going to have one, and there was no point trying to pressurise a resident into doing something he didn't want to do.

I decide to give him a quick wash with a flannel and hot soapy water. Matthew was still quite keen to get on all his clothes before I finish washing him. I had to work quickly.

A quick shave later, a splash of aftershave, and Matthew was ready. I walk him outside the bathroom, and was just about to leave when Matthew alerted me to the final piece of the clothing puzzle.

'Well I need my tie on good sir, can you help me?'

I gently put on Matthew's black and red tie. All dressed in a pin stripe blue and white shirt.

'What do you normally do now then Matthew, do you go to the day centre?'

'Yes, that's right.'

'Do you like it there?'

'Yes, it's quite nice actually.'

'What do you do there?'

'Well not much really, read the newspaper, read a book, that's about it really.'

The day centre was owned by the home. They charged £40 for a half a day, £70 for a full day of activities. The day centre was staffed entirely independently from the home, and no one who already worked for the nursing home was allowed to work in the day centre, according to the rumour spread by the smoking shelter. The rumour was started that the day centre staff actually all got paid more money than the nursing home staff, and didn't want the nursing home staff being 'poached' across to the day centre.

'Anyway sir, I must get on my way, thank you for everything.'

'No problem at all Matthew, nice meeting you.'

I bid my farewells to Matthew and his wife, and walk back up onto the unit. Paul is still by the medication cabinet.

'Thanks for doing that, how did you get on?'

'Well he refused his shower nine times, but apart from that it went well.'

'Honestly, I don't know why we get picked to use all our staff for everything'

'Well, he was getting a little anxious and agitated, even with me in his bathroom.'

'Probably just an excuse mate, they're not dementia units, they're not used to it down there, but you did it, and that's all that matters.'

'Yeah, no problems.'

I go back into the lounge area and continue making the drinks. As a student I would often get into considerable anxiety states as to what sort of mug or beaker each patient would have in the hospitals, and who was diabetic or not. Some of the residents would require small beakers with lids, and others normal plastic mugs. Others just small beakers without lids.

I got all the drinks ready to go on the trolley. Sharon, Katie and Emma were making their way down the corridor to come and help me, and we began distributing the drinks among the residents.

There was a loud bang at the door connecting the lounge area with the other unit. A sprightly lady walked into the lounge area, medium build, short of stature, with bright bobbing blonde hair. It was Sheila the hairdresser. She spoke with a particular bounce in her voice.

'Hello ladies...oh and gentleman I see, who have we got ready then?'

The residents on the unit would get their hair done on a weekly basis, and styled if they preferred. The carers would usually detest any visit from Sheila as she could be quite bossy and assertive with them, and would usually come at a busy time, as they were finishing getting people up, and doing the drinks. There would often be a list in the nursing station of whose hair needed doing. Sometimes Sheila would require a little assistance in getting the residents to her nearby hair salon on the unit, staying with her a few moments, just to help hold a resident's head over the sink.

Sharon immediately shouts out,

'Can you just go and see Jenny, she's in one of the rooms down the right side, I think she knows who is on the list.'

'Right, okay, thank you.'

Sheila walks with great enthusiasm down the corridor. I carry on helping Sharon with the drinks. Sheila walks back into the lounge area, a little more subdued.

'Well I'm not impressed at all, I have basically been told where to go by Jenny.'

Sharon has a quizzical look on her face.

'Why what's up baby?'

'All I wanted to know is who I could take first, and Jenny basically told me she was a 'bit busy at the moment', most rude indeed, and I'm not standing for it.'

Sheila didn't hang around for Sharon to try and speak to her, she simply stormed off the unit. Sharon rolls her eyes.

'Oh my god, here we go again', she laughs, a throaty, crackly laugh.

Sheila would get quite anxious and agitated if she wasn't being helped. It was a constant struggle and battle between the two sides; giving up some time to the hairdresser was seen as one of the more annoying tasks, considering the time of day it used to happen. Sheila was very nice, down to earth lady. When she wanted something to happen, she wanted it to happen instantly, with no back-chat, no arguments, and she would have no qualms in going straight to the top to voice her complaints.

I go over to Andrew to give him his blackcurrant squash. He is looking straight past me, whistling away to himself as he taps his feet. I give him a few sips of his squash, and he immediately tries to grab the beaker off me and tip it upside down. I can feel his immense strength as he tries to fight me with the beaker. He eventually loosens his grip, and I continue to give him a few sips at a time. He starts to put his hand on my leg, and rub it up and down a few times. It starts to become a little unnerving, but the beaker is almost finished, and I stand up quickly, and pop the dirty beaker back on the drinks trolley, ready to be taken down to the kitchen.

Jennifer comes bursting back onto the unit, and walks straight towards Paul, who is sat in the nursing station. Before she gets there, she stops briefly in the middle of the lounge area.

'Right, who has upset Sheila now, own up!'

Sharon laughs.

'Listen Jennifer, it's not fair on these girls, all she was told is that we're very busy at the minute, and she would just have to wait a while. We don't mind helping, it's just very awkward time of the day, you must appreciate that'

'Right, what I don't appreciate is the owner of the home coming to me, saying that Sheila is in tears, and she has threatened to walk out!'

'Oh god, she hasn't has she?'

'Yes, and not for the first time!'

Jennifer walks over to Paul and explains the situation to him.

'Paul, something has to be done about this. It's all getting passed down, straight from the top, and now I am passing it on to you. I think we just need to be a little careful around Sheila, treat her with kid gloves. She is upset, she just wants to do her job. All she wants is one of the carers to help her with some of the residents, taking them back and forth to the salon, it's a few minutes work, so can you speak to everyone and just tell them that?'

'I will. In all fairness to the girls, I do know they get a bit stressed around this time of the morning, and like to get everything finished, all the beds made, and everyone up washed, dressed, and tidy.'

'I know, but we have to be able to work with Sheila. Having the residents' hair done is a part of their weekly routine, and they like having it done, we can't afford to lose Sheila, so we are just going to have to think of a way to work around this.'

'Right.'

'I suggest you nominate one carer, each week, and make it her sole job to work with Sheila in helping her with the residents, so that they can concentrate on getting the people she needs into the salon, whilst the other carers do the drinks and make the beds. This has to be done, I'm not having Sheila keep going to the owner all the time, she has already bitten my head off this morning about it, and I'm not standing for it.'

'Okay, but you do appreciate the stresses these girls are under?'

'I do, I do, but we're going to have to try and make this work, okay? So just make sure you have a word, and sort it. I think Sheila is just trying to calm down a little now, and should be back on your unit a little later, so nominate someone, and let's sort it.'

'Okay.'

Paul nods his head, and Jennifer goes storming back off the unit. Sharon and Katie are huddled in the corner, finishing off the drinks.

'I don't believe it. This isn't the first time you know, she has tried this before, if she doesn't get her own way she goes straight to the top, and it all just cascades back down to us.'

Katie nods.

'Yeah, seems that way alright, I wish I could just do that, and get everything I wanted.'

'You should try it sometime. There's no hierarchy here you know, if you have a problem, go to the owner, then one way or another it will get sorted, and it's out in the open. It's wrong though, you should go to your manager first.'

'Yeah, but nothing ever gets done if you go to Jodie, she just nods in agreement, and then never actions anything, it's a waste of time if you ask me. People should be going to the top, as the hierarchy just doesn't work!'

'Way of the world I'm afraid; in this place, if you don't like something, go right to the top, and then let it all cascade down, until something is done. I've always said though, if you want to complain about anything, always put it in writing, there's no use just gossiping and complaining about things verbally, there's never any evidence. At least if you put something down in writing, that's actual hard evidence.'

'Yeah, not a bad idea really.'

'You've got to baby. If there's anything on your mind, it's the only way forward, but things will never change here. No one is interested, they just turn up for work, do their job, and go home. I think people have truly given up in this place, trying to make a difference, and fighting for what's right, no one gives a toss if we're honest.'

Katie smiles.

'Well it's true love. I'm not one for beating around the bush, you know me, I call a spade a spade, and am proud of the fact. In my day things were very different, and you just had to get on with it.'

Lucy, the frail lady with white hair shouts out from her chair in the lounge.

'Well I don't know do I, I'm I'm I'm I'm I'm I'm I'm I'm...'

Lucy tries to slowly push up with her hands, trying to stand, but half way up, just doesn't have the energy, and sits back down in her seat. She has one eye open, and is still tapping her feet on the floor.

'Thank you Lucy love, she's a sweetie isn't she?' Sharon smiles.

Paul pokes his head into the lounge area.

'Sharon, your daughter's on the phone.'

'Oh? All right love, coming now.'

Sharon had a daughter, and a granddaughter, she doted on both of them, and would be at their beck and call. They would often ring at work at the most inappropriate of times, and with the strangest of requests. These phone calls used to drive some of the other carers mad.

I could see Katie and Emma's faces drop. A split second later, and you would have missed those tiny micro signals that had erupted over their faces. But they were there. I could hear Sharon talking in the nursing station. Her loud voice boomed and travelled down the corridor into the lounge area.

'Right, Okay well I'm a bit busy at the moment, but I'll be there as soon as I can.'

A few moments later and Sharon comes bustling down the corridor.

'Right ladies, my daughter's babysitter has collapsed, and there's no one to look after the baby, so I'm going to sort it out.'

Paul looked a little downbeat.

'Right, well I can't authorise it, so you had best tell Jennifer and sort it out with her.'

'Okay, I will, I'll help finish the drinks off then I'll go, there's no one to look after the baby otherwise. It's either one thing or another isn't it!'

Sharon walked off and started to help out with the drinks once more. I walk back up to Paul. He sighs.

'This isn't the first time something like this has happened you know, I reckon that was a set up, pure and simple.'

'Are you sure?'

'Oh it was planned mate, I'm sure of that, she has done things like this far too often. It's a hard one to call, specially with family matters, but at the end of the day, we can't prove anything, can we?'

'Yeah, it is a hard one to call.'

'There have been countless times when she has called in sick due to her daughter, and her granddaughter, but at the end of the day she has to realise where her loyalties lie, and she's letting the team down all the time. I have heard it all before, I promise you that, I am not even surprised any more.'

Paul walks back into the lounge area and confronts Sharon.

'Do you know if you're coming back at all Sharon? Just in terms of getting cover, you see.'

'I really don't know Paul, I will do my best okay, but I have to sort it out. I'll give you a ring as soon as I know, okay baby?'

'Right, go see Jennifer on your way out, and hopefully they will send someone up to cover you. I'll give the other units a ring.'

'Okay baby, thanks, sorry about this, always something going on isn't there! I'll be back in the manager's office again I am sure, can't get away without sitting in that office these days, I only have to have a sniff of a cold, and I am getting a disciplinary!'

Sharon laughs, a low crackly laugh. There is a hint of light heartedness to her tone.

'I think that's most of the drinks done now, I'm going to go now ladies....and gentleman, I will try to be back as soon as I can, if I can, you will be all right won't you ?'

Katie and Emma nod in agreement.

Sharon asks me to go take a drink to Ella.

'Mind how you go love.'

And with that Sharon walked off confidently down the corridor and out of the unit.

Sharon wouldn't get paid for the time she was off the unit. No one would. No one received any sick pay of any kind, except for statutory sick pay from the government, but that would barely cover any loss of income from a carer's or nurse's wage. The company's strategy was to effectively manage poor attendance, they thought this was best managed by not offering any sick pay to anyone to deter those from throwing a casual 'sickie' or 'duvet day'.

Some of the carers would study the rota, some would go down and photocopy it, without the manager's say so (they would prohibit photocopying of the rota, as it would breach confidentiality, also allowing carers to be able to see exactly who they were working with on each day, which arguably gave them an advantage as to when they would pull the perfect sickie, if they didn't wish to work with certain members of staff). They could also utilise the rota to see when the days were overstaffed, so they could comfortably phone in sick, and keep their conscience clear, knowing that their absence was not putting any undue stress on the team working that day.

The management weren't stupid, despite most of the carers thinking that they were. They would spot these anomalies, and would start to see patterns in people's absences quite clearly. There was never enough proof to comfortably confront anyone about why they were off on particular days. This was not in any way to victimise or try to incriminate honest people about genuine days off; we all got sick from time to time. There would always be people who would try and push the boundaries, and they would always leave a trail. The fact remained that the most common days for anyone to take off would always be:

Days directly preceding or following a bank holiday – Take your pick, either a Thursday or a Tuesday before or after a bank holiday still remained the kings of the days off. Maybe a nursed hangover just required that little extra attention, or an early start down the beer garden. The management would pay particular vigilance to any bank holiday weekends, and keep a close eye on the 'usual culprits'.

Weekends – Not generally both days of a weekend, but a common trick would often be for some of the carers to request a particular weekend day off. They would often have their request refused, and call in sick on the day that they had requested. A total coincidence.

Royal Weddings - We don't tend to have many royal occasions, but the last one resulted in three carers going sick at precisely the same time, on the same day, and they rang within minutes of each other the night before. This caused there to be just one nurse and one carer to try and run a unit with twenty residents. Needless to say, the air was turning blue that day.

World cup - Particular major games, and any match involving England.

Days when there were a strangely higher than average amount of staff on the unit (usually six or more) – This would often result in the unit just merely going down to its usual staffing levels. Any time the unit seemed more staffed than usual, i.e., actually able to run smoothly, someone would call in sick, merely putting it back down to normal levels, every time.

Sickness and Facebook
We didn't have to worry about Facebook prior to 2004. It is increasingly becoming a tool which both nurses and carers have to pay particular attention to. The owner of the home would frequently check on Facebook, and look up new carers and nurses to check on their status or pictures. There was an incident with a nurse not so long ago that had caused him to put that he 'successfully skived a day at work'.

One of the carers read this statement, and reported it to management. That nurse was then in a meeting trying to defend their actions, and had a written warning about the incident. This hadn't helped his case; he was already described as a bit 'flaky', and always going off sick because he felt tired. This was just further evidence that would go against him. One of the carers even helped management by logging into her own Facebook account, letting management look at all the employees' status updates, to see if they could find any further evidence. The carer soon got promoted to a senior carer position.

There were eyes everywhere. And you couldn't trust anyone. Of course, if people were going to go off sick, then they should be aware that Facebook is a tool that can trace your whereabouts if you are foolhardy enough to talk about your each and every move, and potentially share this information with everyone. A further note of caution should be heeded with Facebook's check ins and tagging facilities.

'The NMC issued its guidance in response to a number of nurses being investigated over their social networking activity.'

'The NMC warns that nurses and midwives will put their registration at risk, and students may jeopardise their ability to joint its register, if they:'

- Share confidential information online
- Post inappropriate comments about colleagues or patients
- Use social networking sites to bully or intimidate colleagues
- Pursue personal relationships with patients or service users
- Distribute sexually explicit material
- Use social networking sites in any way that is unlawful

Nursing Times (2011)

> **Pictures**
>
> 'Nurses in particular should be very careful of any pictures of themselves in any compromising situations: drinking alcohol, taking drugs, fornicating. As a nurse you have a professional duty to uphold your profession both in and outside of work. There have been numerous cases brought forward to the NMC regarding nurses and Facebook, some leading to nurses to be struck off the register.'
>
> 'Andy Jaeger, NMC Assistant Director, Professional and Public Communications, and author of the social networking sites advice states 'Most people simply don't realise how much information is shared with the world if you don't adjust your privacy settings on Facebook.'
>
> 'I would advise nurses and midwives to exercise caution when using social networking sites. They could risk their registration if they share sensitive information, make inappropriate comments, or befriend patients online.'
>
> **NHS Your Choice Magazine, Autumn Edition (2011)**

The nurses had put so much pressure onto the management about not being paid any sick pay that the management had to start putting something into place. This was never discussed with any of the carers, and the nurses had received a separate document with their pay packet that detailed what the company was prepared to do. To this day, the carers never knew of this deal that was arranged. The rumour mill had obviously started from somewhere, as many of the carers had asked some of the nurses, out of the blue, if they got paid sick pay. The nurses just said that they were entitled to the same as anyone else, i.e., nothing. That day when the nurses opened their pay packet, they were greeted with an additional piece of paper that stipulated that the company were going to do something about the situation:

The document was described as a protection plan. They were aware that for many of the staff the possibility of being absent from work due to long term sickness or injury is a major worry because of the impact of the loss of pay. You do receive statutory sick pay; however, this is considerably less than the level of income you receive whilst at work. They were offering on a new scheme which entitled staff to receive payment during sickness absence.

Staff with less than one year's service would receive only statutory sick pay, subject to normal rules. For every year of service, the nurses would receive a full month's pay, followed by up to three months' half pay. For every year of experience at the home, this would entitle the nurses to an additional month's full pay.

The nurses had fought hard, and complained, but finally they were being rewarded; there was at least some compensation if they were ever sick. The nurses very rarely went off sick. It was often the carers that would have a worse attendance rate than any of the nurses in the home. The nurses were starting to be a bit more respected in their line of work.

Paul came walking up to me.

'Has Sharon gone now then?'

'Yeah, she has.'

'Let's just watch this space if she returns. She really messes people about at times.'

11-12 p.m.

I walk up the corridor and spot Ella's room on the right. I go in with her mug of blackcurrant squash, and introduce myself.

Ella is a frail old lady with thick brown glasses and a kindly smile. She is wearing a matching brown cardigan and top with brown corduroy trousers. She is half asleep as I walk into her room.

'Hello Ella, I've got a drink for you!'

Ella immediately snaps awake.

'Oh, marvellous, that's absolutely grand that is, please do come and sit down my dear.'

'My name is Jack by the way, I'm a nurse.'

I go and sit on the bed next to Ella. She is immediately brightened up by the presence of me here.

'Ah well, it's like I was saying it should be like that, I mean well, I always thought it would be myself.'

'Ella, I've just got a drink for you.'

'Yes, yes, I know that, but what I mean is I am trying to understand well, what was his name ? He was going to get me something earlier on today'.

Ella was suffering from expressive dysphasia. This can impair a person's speech initiation, general word forming, and articulation. Although people can perfectly understand what is said to them, they have great difficulty communicating their thoughts. It will often come out as a stream of unintelligible sentences.

I notice on the far side of the wall there are a few pictures of Ella with what looks to be her husband, on a pier, and outside a small cottage.

Ella often liked to spend time on her own in her room. Her daughter often said that her mother liked her own company and would while away many hours just sitting in her chair and reading her book or listening to music. Ella had been in the armed services many years ago and had travelled all over the world. She had been diagnosed with vascular dementia a few years ago, and it had become increasingly difficult for her daughter to look after her as she was worried about her falling on her own and becoming so confused she couldn't operate her cooker properly, and was leaving it on as she went to bed. I point to the pictures on the wall.

'Is that you Ella? Where is that Pier ?'

'Oh yes, of course that's me, well I don't know I think it's somewhere in Wales.'

'It looks like Llandudno to me, is it there?' I ask.

'Oh well quite possibly yes, I think it is.' Ella laughs at me.

I gesture towards Ella's mug of blackcurrant squash, and slowly stand up.

'Okay Ella, well I've got your drink there for you, so I shall catch up with you a bit later, okay?'

Ella looks up to me and smiles. I am not sure she has understood what I have just said, but she nods.

'Okay, well yes, you carry on you know, because one day you will have to be in charge of everything you know.'

I thanked her and went on my way. I turned around the corner back to the nursing office. Paul was sat getting files out ready.

'Hi mate, you won't believe this, but we have got a ward round this morning, I've just looked in the diary.'

'Ah right okay, can I be involved in it then?'

'Yeah, sure.'

'I've just been in with Ella, she seems quite a confused lady, does she often keep herself to herself then?'

'Oh don't talk to me about Ella, I've got a few words I need to tell the doctor about her for sure.'

The unit was run by the unit manager, this generally ran pretty smoothly, however there was an overriding manager that would oversee both the unit I was on and the other dementia unit. From time to time this manager would pop upstairs and just check on what had been going on and keep herself up to date. This hardly ever happened; everyone thought it was more of a title rather than an actual job role. But as hierarchy dictated, she would be ultimately responsible for both areas.

One day the unit was incredibly short staffed, so this manager had to fill in upstairs. Paul said when this happened there was usually chaos and a stream of little notes in the daily diary and emails about what needed doing on the unit, which used to rile everyone. On this one occasion the manager filled in upstairs and happened to notice that Ella was sat in her room a lot. She asked the carers if this was Ella's normal presentation. Most agreed, but one carer did seem to think that she was spending more time than normal in her room, despite being perfectly mobile.

Ella would mobilise herself when she wanted to, and would quite often walk up and down the corridor, and come into the lounge area for mealtimes. If you put some old classic Max Bygraves tunes on in the lounge area she would be seen dancing a little and singing along to the tunes. Ella was quite a happy go lucky lady and would do what she wanted, when she wanted. The carers on this particular day must have sounded convincing, as from that one day's assessment, the manager decided that Ella must be put on some Citalopram, an anti-depressant, starting at 20mg once a day. Citalopram would often be used in dementia. Depression was common, but not everyone would require it, it was quite possible to live with dementia and not need an anti-depressant.

Citalopram had its potential side effects, such as nausea, sleepiness, and potential diarrhoea. I am always of the opinion to medicate as least as possible where you can. Medication does have its place but if it is not needed then we should not be giving it.

The manager spoke to the doctor and she got Ella written up for Citalopram to be started straight away. Paul went mad. The manager had made this assessment on the basis of the day and some input of what the carers had told her. In order to clinically judge depression you had to be making these judgements based on observations and changes in presentation over a two week period at least, utilising various depression scales and tools to help.

Ella still ate well at most meal times, still sang and danced in the lounge area and appeared to enjoy herself, she laughed and appeared to be in good spirits. Paul confirmed with the daughter that her mother had always been a solitary lady at times and did like her own company, so Paul felt that Ella was simply misdiagnosed as depressed for what she actually liked doing and was now put on a tablet that she simply didn't need. It wasn't just Paul who disagreed with this decision; three other nurses couldn't believe why she had been put on Citalopram.

When Paul asked Ella herself she was able to state that she wasn't depressed, and her daughter also thought that she wasn't depressed when she came to visit her mother.

What had annoyed Paul even further is that the doctor had completely taken the unit manager's word for it, based on this one day's assumption that she was spending more time in her room.

Paul fought for a long time to get Ella off the anti-depressant. In the ward round they finally agreed to halve the tablet, and to put Ella on 10mg each morning to see if that would have any effect. It was often commonplace not to suddenly stop people's medication, but to gradually titrate them down.

Whilst this was going on Ella was having a lot more falls, and was often found in her room or in the corridor, having fallen for no particular reason. The doctors had agreed at the time that this was probably due to Ella's continuing deterioration in her illness. The decrease in Citalopram continued for a couple of weeks until the next doctors' round where Paul was in charge of it. Paul described the ward round to me; he was also sat in with a consultant who made monthly visits just to have his input on some of our residents that we felt needed another opinion on, as well as the normal doctor who visited, Dr. Edwin. They were all sat round together in the nursing office.

'Hi Paul, so how are things with Ella?'

'Well, at the end of the day, I have spoken to her daughter and she feels she isn't depressed when she comes to visit, she is still eating well, singing and dancing in the lounge area at times, and I don't feel that she is depressed, but she has been having a lot of falls lately.'

'A lot of falls?'

'Yeah, she has been found a few times in her bedroom on the floor, and when I have checked her blood pressure straight afterwards it has been quite low. She hasn't done any serious damage as yet, but the falls do seem to have increased slowly. I think it could just be general deterioration.'

The consultant looks up at Paul and pauses before speaking.

'When did we last review her Citalopram? We reduced it didn't we?'

'Yeh, she is on 10mg now, instead of 20mg, once a day.'

'Why did we reduce the Citalopram?'

'Because she wasn't showing any signs of depression in my mind.'

'But she's now falling, since the reduction of Citalopram?'

'Well yes she is, but I don't think that is attributable, it is probably just coincidental.'

The consultant looks perplexed, and looks over to Dr Edwin.

'I think we should raise the Citalopram back up to 20mg, I'm not happy about these falls.'

'Don't you think its general deterioration?'

'Well it seems that the only change we have made has been the reduction in Citalopram, so let's raise that back up to 20mg, and see where we go from there.'

Paul looked angered, and spoke up.

'Well, I don't think she should be on it at all personally, she's not depressed!'

'It's only a small dosage, and if you said she's falling a lot, I don't want to risk any more falls. I am in agreement with Dr. Edwin, let's put it back up to 20mg and see where we go from there.'

'Right, okay, fine.'

Depression drugs and falls

'Falls are the leading cause of accidental death in the over-65s.'

'Elderly people with dementia are more likely to suffer falls if they are given anti-depressants by care home staff, a study claims.'

'Many dementia patients also suffer from depression and drugs known as selective serotonin uptake inhibitors (SSRIs) are frequently prescribed. But the British Journal of Clinical Pharmacology reports that the risk of injuries from falls was tripled.'

'The Alzheimer's Society called for more research into alternative treatments.'

'The risk of falls following treatment with older anti-depressants is well established, as the medication can cause side effects such as dizziness and unsteadiness.'

'It had been hoped that a move to newer SSRI-type drugs would reduce this problems, but the latest research, from the Erasmus University Medical Centre in Rotterdam, appears to show the reverse.'

'Dr Carolyn Sterke recorded the daily drug use and records of falls in 248 nursing home residents over a two-year period.'

'The average age of the residents was 82, and the records suggested that 152 of them had suffered a total of 683 falls.'

'The consequences of falls were relatively high, with 220 resulting in injuries including hip fractures and other broken bones - and one resident died following a fall.'

'The risk of having an injury-causing fall was three times higher in residents taking SSRIs compared with those not taking the drug, and this risk rose further if the patient was being given sedative drugs as well.'

'Dr Sterke said that these risks needed to be taken into account when assessing whether anti-depressants were required.'

She said: 'Physicians should be cautious in prescribing SSRIs to older people with dementia, even at low doses.'

Professor Clive Ballard, from the Alzheimer's Society, said it was 'worrying' that such a commonly prescribed anti-depressant was causing increased risk.

He said: 'It is important to highlight any aspect of care that might be causing risk to a person with dementia. We want to ensure that people with the condition are always receiving the best care possible.'

'More research is now needed to understand why this anti-depressant is having this effect on people with dementia and if there is an alternative treatment for depression that they could be prescribed.'

'One in three people over 65 will die with dementia yet research into the condition continues to be drastically underfunded. We must invest now.'

BBC News, (2012)

Paul had given up the fight. The doctors had gone full circle on themselves; in the previous ward round they had said that Ella was generally deteriorating and would be falling anyway due to the progression of her illness, and now they were trying to attribute the falls to the drop in Citalopram. Paul had lost the will, he had battled for months to get Ella off this drug, and now just when he thought he was getting somewhere they had put it back up to its original dosage, despite everything he had been saying about Ella not being depressed. He rang the daughter immediately after the ward round and explained what the doctors had decided to do. She also wasn't happy with the decision, but everyone felt they had to go along with it.

As nurses we are supposed to be advocates for people who cannot have their own say any more in their health and wellbeing, and we are supposed to be fighting for the best treatment. What I learned at university about depression obviously hadn't seemed quite correct; apparently you could get prescribed anti-depressants, even if you were not depressed. If you liked your own company for a few hours a day that was tantamount to depression, it would seem.

Paul was so mad that when he was doing Ella's care plan for mental health, he wrote a full blown account of why he thought that Ella should not be on Citalopram, describing her daily routine and how she was still eating and drinking and enjoying leisure time in the lounge area by singing and dancing. In his opinion, he wrote in the evaluation, we should be making steps to reducing and eventually coming off the Citalopram. He even put Ella's daughter's views within the care plan and Ella's.

A few days later, the care plan disappeared. Vanished, and a new care plan had been replaced, without Paul's original wording. He was shocked. He tried desperately to find the original care plan that he had wrote. There was no way he thought that the doctors could argue next time about keeping her on the drug, but it had gone, never to be found again. From that day onwards Paul never trusted the unit manager again. There was no way to prove whether the care plan had simply been discarded by mistake, but it was so well written and had a wealth of evidence based practice behind it, that Paul was suspicious that it had gone missing because people hadn't liked what he had to say.

Paul had felt completely powerless, and fed up with the hierarchy of 'power', he felt he couldn't make a difference any more and that the resistance was too much. He didn't seem to have a say in the residents' care, and if he did it wouldn't be listened to.

I sat stunned by what Paul had said to me. Having just been in to see Ella myself, I simply wouldn't have made that judgement at all about her being depressed; maybe I had learned something at university after all.

'Yeah, amazing story, isn't it?' Paul whispered.

'Sure is, so what's the plan today then, to try and get her off it again?'

'I'm just not going to bother now any more. I have had my battles with the doctors, and they just don't want to listen to me. I am obviously not looking out for Ella's best interests, and my thirty years experience on the wards simply doesn't seem to count for anything.'

'Oh it definitely should do!'

'Well, as I said to you, it doesn't seem to in this case; they would rather listen to a manager who is barely up here for a day!'

'Crumbs.'

'Yeah, a terrible state of affairs, you better watch yourself, that's all I'm going to say.'

As if she had heard exactly what we were discussing, Ella at this present moment in time started to walk past the nursing office with a bright grin on her face. Paul shouted out to her.

'Hello Ella, how are ya?'

Ella initially couldn't work out where the sound was coming from, and then turned towards Paul. Her eyes lit up and a big smile erupted over her face.

'Ah, you see, I thought I would get away with that! I was just testing you there,' she laughed.

'Ella! I would never forget you, don't be silly! You going to get some lunch in a bit, are you?'

'Oooh yes that would be lovely, where will that be then?'

'Just in the lounge, keep heading down that way, but it won't be for a while yet, although there is some music playing in the lounge I do believe, go and see the girls, they will sort you out.'

'Ooh, fantastic, right-o, well I can't stop and chat all day, I have to go and err, do some things, you know.'

'Okay Ella, catch you later!' Paul exclaimed.

And with that Ella walks off merrily towards the lounge area, greeting other residents as she slowly walks into the lounge.

'She's a smasher, she really is,' Paul says.

'Sadly, completely puddled though,' he adds.

She was a very chirpy lady, and seemed very bubbly. I would have to prepare myself more than I realised; it seemed that doctor's rounds were still going to be quite a challenge.

Outside the building, in the car park, there was a screech of tyre rubber as a large gleaming black BMW 5 series parks up, crossing boldly over two spaces. The number plate reads GRE 74. The car engine switches off abruptly and the driver's door opens. There is a slight squeak as the highly polished black leather shoes touch the glistening tarmac. These are Dr. Greeta's shoes.

Dr. Greeta was dressed in an immaculate pin stripe grey suit. He had an immaculately shaven baby face, of Indian origin, and with jet black short hair, with piercing green eyes. He was of medium build, but carried an air of authority that was unsurpassed. He clutched a thick black leather briefcase. He reached into his pocket and took out his phone to check for his messages, ruffling back his shirt to reveal an immaculate Breitling watch. He delved further into his pocket and reached for his Iphone. He punched in a few numbers and began phoning.

'Nicky, yes I'm here at the home, remind me again who I am going to see at my 3 p.m. appointment please.'

There was a brief silence for a few moments. Dr. Greeta stood patiently. A few more moments passed, and Dr. Greeta smiled to himself.

'Excellent, thank you Nicky, I'll catch up with you later.'

Dr. Greeta punched a button on his key fob, and the BMW clicked and clunked solidly. He began walking towards the reception area of the home. The receptionist smiled to him as he walked past. Dr. Greeta didn't need to sign in like everyone else in the home; the receptionist did that for him. Dr. Greeta was well respected amongst his peers, and he was often chairing conferences and lecturing on psychiatry. He was a psychiatrist specialising in dementia care, and despite the youthful looks he had been doing this job for around twenty years. He took everything in his stride. Sometimes you could barely hear his voice as it was so softly spoken and dulcet. He was so calm and collected, and you hung upon his every word. People who went to his lectures described his words as silky smooth and dripping with enthusiasm and intellect.

Just as Dr. Greeta was making his way up the stairs, there was another, different sounding screech of tyres in the car park. A clunky, clattery type sound. A large Audi estate car, looking a little worse for wear was making its way slowly into the car park, and parked up carefully in the parking bay. The car door opens.

Dr. Edwin steps out onto the tarmac. He is dressed in casual light beige chinos, and a red and white striped shirt. He has small black framed glasses, and a receding hairline. He has a goofy, yet winsome grin. He is wearing a dark brown rucksack, and slowly starts to make his way towards the reception area. Dr. Edwin does have to sign in. He is not a consultant, but the resident GP; it would take some time, authority and experience behind him until he would be signed in by the reception girl. Dr. Edwin specialised in dermatology, but he did know enough about psychiatry to offer helpful and friendly advice. He was always willing to go the extra mile for our residents, and whilst he did not necessarily have the charm or charisma of Dr. Greeta, he was still respected in his field, and an invaluable asset for the home. Dr. Edwin was your bumbling Hugh Grant to Dr. Greeta's smooth George Clooney.

Dr. Edwin finishes signing in, and walks up the stairs. He bumps into Dr. Greeta just before they get to the door of the unit.

'Hey, how's it going ?' Dr. Greeta asks Dr. Edwin.

'Yeah, fine thanks, how about you, hey did you get the phone you wanted in the end?'

Dr. Greeta smiles, reaches into his pocket, and pulls out his shiny new Iphone and shows it to Dr. Edwin.

'Oh you bastard!'

'You still running 3GS?'

'Yeah afraid so, it will be another few months till I get a look at that bad boy, how's the screen on that thing?'

Dr. Greeta lights up his Iphone and it dazzles with its brightness. He aims it at Dr Edwin's eye line. Dr. Edwin smiles.

'Wow, pretty impressive. I can't wait to get my hands on one, can you still check all your EMIS clients on there ?'

Dr. Greeta smiles, a half smile.

'Yeah, the company don't like me doing it without a secure network, but it's smooth to operate, and I can diagnose on the move now! Technology hey, utterly fantastic, it's made a massive difference to the way I work.'

'Oh yeah, for sure, well for now us lowly doctors are still using 3GS, but hey, I'll get there one day.'

Dr. Greeta smirks, and puts his phone back into his pocket. Greeta and Edwin worked well together, but Greeta always seemed to have the upper hand in everything: cars, phones, houses. Edwin was always one step behind.

Dr. Greeta punches the code in for Franklyn unit, and the two doctors walk through the double doors.

Bob is walking up the corridor, salivating profusely. He walks straight past Dr. Greeta and Edwin, mumbling to himself under his breath.

The two doctors walk to the nursing office. Paul greets both of them, and introduces them to me. Greeta gives a me a smirk as he looks down at me. The nursing office is so cramped that Paul has to go and get a rather small green bucket from the lounge area and turn it upside down in the nursing office. I stand awkwardly in the corner, and Paul sits uncomfortably next to me perched on the small green bin. Greeta sits in prime position on the main office chair, and Edwin sits next to him on the only other chair in the office. Greeta taps away on the computer and logs into his own private network. A horde of numbers and random letters appear up on the screen, and important looking warnings flash up every few seconds. He spins round on his chair, and begins the ward round.

'Right, who are we here to see?'

Paul coughs a nervous cough.

'Daniel needs a medication review'

Daniel had been having a considerable amount of falls recently, and was becoming a little verbally aggressive and agitated at times. He was on Risperidone, which was an antipsychotic, and the only antipsychotic licensed for treatment of dementia related behavioural disturbances. There was some considerable debate about the drug's efficacy in dementia, and one of the main side effects of the drug was an increase in the risk of having a stroke, as well as the usual side effects of feeling drowsy, and ironically could cause an increase in agitation itself. It was often a mine field prescribing drugs, and not everyone would fit a perfect pattern of behaviour, or react to drugs in defined neat little ways.

A report had been published looking into the efficacy of anti psychotic medication and its use in dementia.

The Banerjee report, published in 2009, was a highly controversial report that detailed the evidence behind the use of these anti psychotics, and how much of a difference they made to people with dementia. Published by the Department of Health, it is readily available on the internet for anyone to peruse at their leisure. What they were specifically *not* supposed to be prescribed for was to curb or stop behavioural and psychological symptoms of dementia (BPSD).

BPSD would incorporate such areas as wandering, some behaviour, agitation, restlessness, and aggression. These were all symptoms that Daniel displayed on a daily basis. His wife would often visit and get a little upset about the amount of falls he was having, so initially the doctors reduced Daniel's

Risperidone, to see if that had any form of affect at all. It didn't seem to. So they put the Risperidone back up. You would often be in a very difficult position as a doctor, trying to do your best for the resident, but sometimes small changes in medication, or even large ones, didn't seem to have any noticeable effect. Daniel was currently prescribed Risperidone in dispersible form, so that it would disperse on his tongue and dissolve naturally. He was currently on 500mcg tablet in the morning, and two 500mcg tablets in the evening. Daniel had to be prescribed these orodispersible forms as the previous incarnations of the tablet he would frequently chew, spit back at you, and tell you to fuck off.

Anti psychotic medication

Taken from: The use of anti psychotic medication for people with dementia: Time for action report, Banerjee,(2009):

- 'An analysis should be made of whether the behaviour (e.g. reversal of sleep-wake cycle so that the person with dementia is awake at night) is a problem primarily for the person with dementia, or for their carers'
- 'Where intervention is needed, psychological approaches such as structured social interaction should be used in the first instance'
- 'The medication should be used at the lowest possible effective dose, for the shortest possible time, ideally less than 12 weeks.'

'Current systems appear to deliver a largely anti psychotic based response, and it is clear that these medications are being prescribed to deal with behavioural and psychological symptoms in dementia rather than just for psychosis.'

'As with all medication, anti psychotics can have considerable side effects. Most notably:'

- Rigidity
- Persistent muscle spasms
- Tremors
- Restlessness

'Primarily anti psychotics in dementia are used to treat restlessness, aggression and psychiatric symptoms in people with dementia.'

'There is no evidence that these drugs improve restlessness or other non-aggressive behavioural symptoms (Schneider, 2006). Up to a quarter of people with dementia in the UK may be on anti psychotics at any time. This equates to 180,000 people with dementia being treated with anti psychotic medication by the NHS.'

'The large majority of the medications will be prescribed by GP's, with a strong suggestion that people with dementia in care homes may be at particular risk (Banerjee, 2009).'

'If, at any one time, we are treating approximately 180,000 people with dementia with anti psychotic medication in any year, and we make the conservative assumption that the average treatment episode is the 6-12 weeks used in trials, this equates to the following:

- An additional 1,800 deaths per year; and
- An additional 1,620 CVAEs (cerebrovascular adverse events), around half of which may be severe.'

Banerjee, (2009)

Daniel's medication had to be reviewed every six weeks. This was best practice in order to assess whether or not the drug was working efficiently, or the amount prescribed needed to be altered.

He had still been found on many occasion lying down on his floor, or any floor in the unit. His wife had not noticed any change in his behaviour since his Risperidone had been increased; he was still wandering, agitated, and restless at times, and he would still be a little verbally aggressive.

Greeta listened intently as Paul explained all of this, nodding at times.

'What would you like to do then, do you think the Risperidone needs reducing then?'

Paul nodded.

'I would, I mean personally I would take him off it all together, because I don't think it is doing any good at all.'

Edwin cleared his throat.

'Well I don't think it would be a good idea to take him off it all together, but we can certainly look at maybe reducing the dose at tea time.' It was usually never good practice to suddenly stop taking medications; they would usually titrate you off a given drug slowly and surely, so they could monitor the effects.

'What do you think Dr. Greeta?'

Greeta, looked up at Edwin, and then at Paul. He appeared a little unsure. Having recently qualified I felt quite confident with my up to date knowledge of current licensing and medication in dementia, so I decided to give my opinion.

'Shouldn't we be looking to reduce the Risperidone anyway, what with the Banerjee report? We can't use the medication just to stop Daniel wandering surely?'

Edwin turned to me.

'Well, that is true, but we are talking end stage dementia here, and anti-psychotics I feel do have a place.'

I decide to continue with my point.

'Plus, I have always been told that there is not much of an evidence base for them anyway within dementia, and their efficacy is dubious.'

Dr. Edwin didn't look particularly impressed.

'Well Mr Banerjee hates all anti-psychotics, that is for certain, but evidence base is fine, but I have seen them do wonders with people here, and all over, it's all very well having reports for everything.'

Reports usually took many months, sometimes years, to collate information and strive for the evidence base, working closely with patients and professionals, to document a drug's efficacy. As a university student you were constantly being told to read reports, and make sure everything you documented in an assignment was backed up with evidence. There was even a module that we had to endure entitled evidence based practice. It was one of the cornerstones and gold standard of your nurse training. You couldn't just argue or debate against anything that didn't have a solid grounding in fact and research.

Dr. Greeta looked up at me.

'Well, let's just reduce the tea time dose to 500mcg, and see.'

'Okay' I stammer. I had felt pleased that I asserted what I wanted to say, but still felt a hot sweat come over my brow as I stared back at Greeta and Edwin, who were now both looking towards Paul in an anticipatory silence.

'I agree, let's not fiddle around with it for at least a few weeks though, we need enough time to see if it will have any effect or not,' Paul stated clearly.

Dr. Greeta and Dr. Edwin nodded. Edwin was passed over the folder containing all the medication sheets for everyone, and quickly documented the change in medication to be set at one 500mcg tablet in the morning, and one in the evening. He signed the change.

The medication sheets (or marrs sheets) had to be signed off by a doctor for any change in medication. We as nurses could not sign for any changes. The sheets were frequently altered by a lot of the nurses, mainly the unit manager; they were crossed out and changed without any official say so. These would often be medications such as Lactulose or Movicol (to help bowel function). For example, if the medication sheet stated 'Once a day, as required', there would be a line crossed through the 'as required' and marked in black ink would be 'please give daily'. If a doctor had not authorised these changes, then this was technically illegal. Unless you were a nurse prescriber, you are not in a position to change people's medications. If medications needed changing, then they needed to be discussed with the doctor, and signed off by them.

Dr. Greeta stood up, calmly and securely. You could almost eat the tension in the air. Dr. Greeta, being a consultant, didn't have to stay for the whole of the ward round, he would only ever see a maximum of three people in his consultations, and he would see up to three people once a month. He said his goodbyes, and walked calmly off the unit, clutching his briefcase solidly.

'And what are we doing about Daniel's pain relief at present ?' Paul asked.

'What's he on at the moment then?'

'He is on two co-codamols, four times a day. I was just wondering if it might be better for him to be on a low dose matrifen patch?'

Dr. Edwin shuffled in his seat a little, and looked down at his shoes, and mumbled to himself.

'Well...I shouldn't tell you this..but I'm going to anyway. The cost of putting him on a matrifen patch will far outweigh co-codamol at present, it's something like £30 a month to have him on a patch, as opposed to just £5-£10 for co-codamol. If he's taking that okay then I would just leave it for now.'

Paul frowned a little.

'Whatever you think doctor, just a suggestion.'

The specific cost for a box of ten matrifen 12mcg patches, to cover a month's supply (as one is given every 72 hours) would work out to around £37.70 for the month. Co-codamol cost £11.24 for a month's supply.

Edwin continued to stay in the nursing office, and Paul started to go through the list of people to discuss on the unit. The ward round sheet would slowly be added to on a weekly basis, documenting any changes or areas of concern that you would wish the doctor to look at or discuss. The ward rounds were split, so you would never have to discuss all twenty patients each week. The way in which the residents were to be discussed (other than if there was a particular concern about a resident) were based upon the GSF, the Gold Standards Framework.

This was an evidence based approach, optimising the care of residents nearing the end of life, a grading or scoring system which would help define how often a doctor was required to see someone based upon their condition and GSF status. Graded from A-D, residents would be evaluated each month and re-graded if necessary. We are always trying to work towards the best interests of people in our care, and using a guidance such as the GSF allows us to provide better care as they approach the end of their lives. It is utilised to provide and improve a prediction of need for support.

Gold standards framework coding

A – 'All' – Stable
Years + prognosis

B – 'Benefits' – Unstable / frequent exacerbations
Months prognosis

C – 'Continuing care' – deteriorating
Weeks prognosis

D – 'Days' – Dying / terminal phase
Days prognosis

Gold standards framework centre, (2005)

If a resident was graded C or D, then that resident would be seen by a doctor every single week. If a resident was a category A, then they would not be seen as often, however everyone on this unit was seen at least every two weeks regardless. This would have implications if there was a death of a resident at any given time. If a resident had suddenly died, and they had not been seen by a doctor in over two weeks, then this would warrant an autopsy to clearly define the cause of death, even if the death was expected or not (these residents were all in the 'expected death' category). So it was incredibly important that the doctor saw everyone, and regularly. You wouldn't want to explain to a grieving relative that their husband or wife was about to be autopsied due to a simple clerical error.

'I think we need to look at reducing Ella's Citalopram again, she's currently on 20mg, and she is still singing and dancing at times in the lounge area, and eating and drinking well. Her daughter is not noticing any changes in her mood, and she is being sociable at times'

Dr. Edwin scratches his head a little.

'Now we put this back up to 20mg already didn't we, because we were worried about her falls weren't we?'

'Yes, that's right. I didn't personally agree with the decision, because she was deteriorating anyway, and having some falls. I just don't think we need to have her on a drug that she doesn't need.'

Dr. Edwin scratches his head a little more.

'I see where you're coming from, but it's only a small dose, and it's not going to hurt her, but maybe we could try 10mg for now and see. I don't really want to mess around too much with the drug, because when we took her off it last time it was a disaster.'

Paul looked pleased with a 'semi win', for his resident.

'Okay, let's halve the dose and see where we go from there then.'

It wasn't always easy to try and state your beliefs and medication you thought a resident should be on; whilst the nursing team were advocates for the resident, it was ultimately the doctor's decision.

The doctors could only really go on what the nursing team communicated to them, and then ultimately they had to make their own clinical judgement. Paul would often say to me that the process was a juggling act at times and could be incredibly difficult to get right. He would feel beaten and trodden on in some of the decisions that were ultimately made, and particularly with Ella, it had felt like one big struggle to fight for her and be her advocate in her medication regime.

I had sat in on many ward rounds during my student nursing days, and they could be difficult and challenging. Everyone was just trying to do their best for the patient. There was never any malice in the ward rounds that I had attended, but it had sometimes seemed that doctors would make very quick and irrational decisions based more upon controlling the patient's behaviour, rather than looking at other non medical interventions.

Medicine was always supposed to be the last resort. I lost count of the times where students were shot down in anything they tried to advocate because the 'lecture room was not the real world'. It appeared to be a universal damnation and served to highlight that there was still clearly a practice gap between education and the clinical environment. A gap which would always remain, no matter how much education changed. In order to get a balance, both areas should be working together in harmony, but that wasn't always easy, and not everyone was always going to be on the same page. As a student I had felt highly dejected and unmotivated by many of the nurses I had worked with, with their morals beaten, hiding behind a sea of paperwork, and spending less and less time with the people that matter the most, the patients.

I observed as Paul went through the rest of the residents on his list. There wasn't anything else major to discuss, the usual smattering of suspected UTI's and chest infections, which were all very common with the elderly. There would be considerable debate on whether to treat or not, particularly with chest infections. Chest infections could be a common cause of eventual death with the elderly, so whether to treat or not was a hot topic.

As you are acting within the best interests of your resident, you would normally treat with some antibiotics, but a lot of relatives would see a chest infection as a natural sign that the end could be near. If the doctor or the nursing team thought that the resident was in any amount of pain from such an infection, then they would treat it immediately. If the resident did not show any signs of pain, the doctors wouldn't always prescribe antibiotics, and would continue to monitor and observe.

Every single one of the residents here on the unit was not for resuscitation. The most important thing was to make sure they were not in any pain. A resistance can be built up to antibiotics, so sometimes being over cautious and carefree with prescribing could in fact be just as bad as not being cautious.

The same would occur with urine infections. Most commonly, the doctor would advise to push fluids for a few days, and encourage more fluid input, rather than go straight for the antibiotics. Other times it was deemed necessary to start the antibiotics straight away.

Dr. Edwin had packed up his own black bag, and was off to the other unit. Paul continued to sit in the office. He now had to update every resident that had been discussed on their individual files, to say that they had been seen and discussed by the doctor, and the changes, if any, that had been made.

Katie comes sauntering up the unit and pops her head round to the nursing office.

'You okay in here? Jack, are you going to be all right to help feed in a moment? We're just getting lunch ready.'

'Yeah, fine, no problem.'

Emma comes around the corner from the other side of the corridor, and also pokes her head through to the nursing office.

'Just to let you know, Daniel's lying down in the middle of the corridor, and he's taken his pad off, and his pants and trousers. We could probably do with moving him for lunch.'

She pauses a short while, and glances back behind her.

'He's sat on the radiator...and he's going to the toilet.'

12–1 p.m.

I can hear Sharon's loud voice booming down the corridor, talking to some of the residents.

'Yes, I'm back, panic over!'

Sharon pops her coat back in the store cupboard, and walks back into the lounge area as though nothing had happened.

'Panic over everyone, Sharon is back! Right, what needs to be done then?'

It was time to start getting some of the residents to the table and ready for lunch. Each resident is given a cloth bib to protect their clothes and dignity. Most residents welcome these, but others would tear them off as soon as you put one round them. Each of the staff members wore thin plastic white aprons for all mealtimes.

Sharon and Katie were now busying themselves around the kitchen area, preparing trays for residents who were still in the corridors, getting beakers of squash ready and various cutlery. Sharon beckons over to me.

'Can you just walk Elsie over to the table please love, ready for dinner?'

'Sure thing.'

Most people would be taken to the table, to encourage a sense of familiarity and routine. Sharon would often whisk people to the table without asking them, or rather she would tell them they needed to go to the table. I would often ask residents where they would like to sit. This wasn't always possible, and they wouldn't always be able to give you an answer, but there would always be residents that could tell you.

Paul would have frequent battles with Sharon over this. One evening he was talking to a resident who was sat in her chair in the lounge area. The conversation went as follows:

'Is it time to go for tea yet Paul?'

'Not yet my dear, in about half an hour or so.'

'Oh right okay love, does that mean I have to go and sit at the table then?'

'You can sit wherever you like, if you want to sit here and have your tea that's fine with me, it's your choice, just remember it's up to you.'

'Oh all right love, can I really sit here and have my tea?'

'Of course you can, just make sure no one tries to make you do things you don't want to do. It's entirely up to you, just see how you feel.'

'Okay love, thank you.'

Paul returned to the lounge area about half an hour later, and sure enough, the resident was whipped away to the table, and sat with the other residents.

Elsie was sat in one of the main chairs in the centre of the lounge, looking a little flat in mood. She had a walking frame, but required some assistance in order to stand up. I walked over to her and gently helped lift her up onto her frame, and she began slowly walking with the frame with me by her side.

'Is there any room at the table?'

'Yes, plenty of room, where would you like to sit?'

Elsie pointed to a table that already had three other lady residents on it: Donna, Jilly, and Mindy.

We slowly walk over to the table, and I gently sit Elsie onto the chair and push her in so she is right up close to the table.

Mindy glances up and smiles at me. Mindy was deaf, but she could understand basic simple commands and could lip read if you spoke clearly and faced her fully. She had short black hair, and small wire frame glasses. Her front teeth were missing, but she could still speak to you in a semi Welsh accent.

One night shift, Mindy had gone to bed. She wouldn't normally let anyone get her changed or ready for bed as she got a little paranoid about people trying to 'steal' her clothes from her, and she was frightened that she would never get them back. Mindy had shut the door to her room, and somehow was able to work out how to lock the door from the inside. Every door had this facility but the residents were usually unable to work out how to lock the door as it required a specific knack to it. Ordinarily this wouldn't be a problem as there were back up keys to each and every room.

Paul had rushed to the nursing office, got a spare key to the room, and came back to unlock the door. After much fiddling around with the key, it seemed unresponsive and wasn't turning as it should. Eventually the key snapped off in the keyhole. Paul frantically tried again knocking on the door, hitting it as hard as he could, and shouting out to Mindy.

Through a tiny crack in the door Paul was able to briefly see an outline of Mindy who was clearly in bed. He could hear some faint snoring emanating from her bedroom. She was fast asleep. Paul had a locked door, a broken key in the lock, and a deaf resident to contend with.

Paul tried frantically to open the door but to no avail. He rang to the other nurses on duty and they couldn't get the door open either, or the spare key to move in the door. Paul started sweating profusely and started to panic that if there was a fire, there would be no way to get Mindy out safely.

There was only one thing for it. After ringing the manager of the unit and waking her up at around midnight, she concurred that the best thing to do would be to ring the handyman.

Derek the handyman was a cool confident twenty something with razor short hair and a physique to match a men's health model. All the younger female carers in the home fancied him, and some would blush at his mere presence. He was a 'man's man'. Nothing was too difficult a task for him. He was married, with two children, but that hadn't stopped him from sleeping with two of the carers, one receptionist, and a nurse since he had started working here. He used to say he was going off on 'errands' some afternoons. His errands consisted of picking carers up on their days off and sleeping with them in his car on top of a hill.

Paul sat patiently in the office area. Around ten minutes later there was a click of the unit door and there was Derek, ready and waiting to sort the problem out.

'Ah thank God your here. I don't know what to do about this situation, but obviously we need this door open.'

'Yeah no problem Paul, I think we can sort it. Where is it then?'

Paul ushered Derek to Mindy's door. Derek had a quick fiddle of the key inside the lock and gave the door a couple of hard shakes. He kept muttering 'right' under his breath, as he studied all aspects of the wooden frame. Paul was standing silently beside him.

'I don't know if the fire service needs calling for anything like this? I don't know where we go from here really, we obviously need the door open.'

Derek took one look at Paul, and smiled.

'Nah, they won't do anything, we will get this open don't worry. Can you just hold onto the door handle really tightly for me?'

'Okay.'

Derek took a few good paces back from the door, looking at it square on. Paul was holding onto the handle for dear life, not sure exactly what Derek was planning, but realisation soon crept over him.

Derek gave one last command to Paul.

'Right Paul, now don't move your hands whatever you do.'

'Okay.'

Derek walked back as far as he could to the far side of the corridor, made a few short sharp bursts forward with his legs, raised his right leg up high and channelled his right foot straight into the door. A large cracking noise rippled through the corridor, and the door frame shook. Paul was holding on tightly. Derek moved back again for another kick, this time more forceful than the last. He threw his right foot into the door once more, and even more cracking sounds erupted. There was a quick popping and the door flew open. Paul instinctively let go of the door handle. The door crashed into the wall in Mindy's room. Mindy was still fast asleep, completely oblivious to the gallant attempt at rescuing her from potential danger. Derek smiled to himself and looked at the large crack on the remaining part of the door.

'Mick will probably kill me for that, but it had to be done, we couldn't risk it; if there was a fire, we would never have got her out.'

Paul felt a little deflated. Derek smiled at Paul.

'Okay Paul mate, see you in the morning!'

'Cheers Derek, you're a lifesaver.'

'No problem at all, all part of the service.'

And with that Derek walked off the unit, as calm as anything, all in a day's (or night's) work.

Here at the table this afternoon Mindy was starting to look a little agitated as she looked at me.

'Where's mine?' Mindy shouted out.

Mindy wasn't always diplomatic, and would often shout her orders. I mouth the word 'soon' as best I can, and Mindy appears to understand me. One of the carers had recently bought in a small whiteboard to use for her as she could also understand basic words if they were written large and clearly.

The whiteboard worked well, but sometimes if the carers were a little rushed it seemed that this would get missed sometimes and Mindy would just be plated up a meal that she would most probably want to eat anyway. I often felt this was a stress that I would come to feel everywhere. As a student it was always a constant battle to spend time with residents, and it seemed such a shame that a few precious minutes were sometimes all you had with someone on a daily basis. The daily tasks and duties of a nurse and care assistant seemed to eat into most of the day, leaving very little time to spend with who you were caring for.

A typical day in nursing	
8.00 – 8.25	Handover
8.25 – 8.45	Phoning all units to chase up an agency worker from agency. Eventually rang agency and found worker had been 'pinched' for another unit, now on Melvin.
8.45 – 10.15	Morning Medication round **(1hr 30mins)**
	Phone call relative
	Spending 10 minutes with AA having a chat
	Spending 5 minutes with BB having a chat
	Spending 2 minutes with CC having a chat
10.15 – 10.30	Drinks preparation
10.30 – 10.40	Serving drinks
10.40 – 12.21	Ward round – Dr Edwin
12.21 – 12.41	**AM BREAK**
12.41 – 13.10	Updating orange doctor's notes in all files
13.10 – 13.56	Lunch Time Medication round **(46 minutes)**
13.56 – 14.18	SALT referral for DD
	Showing new cleaner down onto another unit
	Assisting AA on the toilet and walking to chair

14.18 – 14.28	Phone call – relative – Update on DD
14.28 – 14.35	Discussion with handyman about allotted gloves / wipes
14.35 – 14.51	Logging onto computer – starting handover template and updating residents' changes from ward round
14.51 – 14.53	Writing daily work sheet for next day
14.53 – 14.58	Discussion with carers on importance of updating bowels charts as not being filled in
14.58 – 15.00	Phone call – relative – Update on AA
15.00 – 15.02	Cup of tea / small discussion with relative
15.03 – 15.33	**LUNCH**
15.33 – 16.50	Daily nursing notes x 20 Phone call – relative Phone Call – relative (to see how her daughter was after speaking to her)
16.50 – 16.52	Cup of tea
16.52 – 17.12	**PM BREAK**
17.12 – 18.50	Teatime Medication round **(1hr 38 mins)** (including feeding one resident)
18.50 – 19.17	Clerking in medication for supplier delivery Phone call – relative – Update on FF Phone Call – relative – Update on GG

19:05	Talking to relative to say not coming in to visit
19:25	Checking 2 x Matrifen patches with Manager
	Phone Call – Agency – update if needing any staff
19.17 – 19.38	Finalising handover
19.38 – 19.42	Going downstairs to printer for handover
19.42 – 20.00	Chat with carers; small debrief
20.00 – 20.20	Handover with night staff

Approximate resident contact time = 20 minutes

Jilly wore two hearing aids, which she would often complain weren't working. She suffered from a lot of anxiety, and would often ask for pills to 'perk her up', and had considerable anxiety about being incontinent, despite wearing daily incontinence pads. Jilly waves towards me and shouts out.

'Love, I need to speak to you please.'

'Okay, what's the matter Jilly?'

'Well, I think I've wet my pad you see, and I am worried about it.'

'Jilly you will be fine, you were just taken to the toilet. Sharon took you a few minutes ago'

'Are you sure love? Have I got a thick pad on? - Because I am worried that I will wee myself otherwise.'

'Yes, honestly, and we can take you again after lunch. Don't worry, you have the thickest pad we could find on, so you don't have to worry about that, that is what they are for, they will absorb anything.'

'Honestly?'

'Honestly.'

'Oh, okay, then love, sorry to bother you, my memory is terrible at times.'

Jilly smiled at me, and seemed more content. This would be a daily behaviour trait of Jilly's, but if you could just reassure her and give her a bit of attention then she would become a lot more relaxed.

Donna was sat at the table in her wheelchair, also looking quite anxious.

'Hey, Jack.'

'Jack, I want to speak to you, you see that man over there?'

I look to where Donna is pointing. Bob is asleep in his chair on the far side of the lounge.

'Well he fell over the other day, and I just wanted to know if he was all right.'

'Oh he's fine yes, he was just walking around today, no problems.'
'Oh good, because I was worrying about him all night you see, so I am glad he is okay.'
'Yep, no problems at all, don't worry. I'm going to get you some lunch in a minute.'
'Not too much though, because I have a dentist's appointment in a few days and I don't want to spoil my teeth.'
'Just eat what you can Donna.'
'Will do.'

And with that Donna gives me a salute, and starts laughing, a wheezy, deep laugh, which seems to go on for several moments.

There is a loud rattle and clanking coming from afar. This is the food trolley being wheeled down the corridor and into the lounge area. The food was brought up every mealtime in the Bain Marie, with piping hot food in each of its storage areas. The kitchen staff bought this up anywhere between about 12.15 p.m. – 12.30 p.m. It was being brought up by a small framed girl with blondish hair tied back into a pony tail. She didn't say much, simply wheeled it in and let Sharon take hold of it.

'Thanks, baby.'

The girl walked off back down the corridor. Sharon pulled a face as she turned. I walk over to Sharon.

'Did you hear what they said about her?'

'What's that?'

'They couldn't find her for ages in the kitchen, and the rumour goes that she was snorting cocaine in the cupboard, but they couldn't find any evidence of it, and so they are still letting her work here.'

'What?' I say in disbelief.

'Honestly, it's true, for hours they couldn't find her, and when they did she was acting very strangely indeed, but there was no evidence to pin on her, so she is still working, I don't trust her myself though, she's a very quiet girl, but it just goes to show you doesn't it?'

The quiet girl is Suzie, only nineteen years of age. She had been working for the company for just a few months. Her job was simple: to help transport all the food when it was ready up to the units, on time. One day she turned up looking a bit bedraggled and a bit tired under the eyes. The kitchen staff thought nothing of it, and just assumed she had been partying the night before. Suzie had done her usual routine in the morning, and taken all the hot food up to each unit, one by one. She had returned back down to the kitchen area, and promptly gone on her break. Twenty minutes had passed, then thirty.

The kitchen staff were starting to get a little suspicious. They sent one of their staff out to go and locate Suzie. She was nowhere in sight; she wasn't at the smoking shelter, nor was she talking to the laundry ladies. They found Suzie over an hour later, round the back of the kitchen area, in a store cupboard sat upright on a small stool, fast asleep, her nostrils inflamed, and when she woke to the kitchen manager her eyes were completely bloodshot and she was very excitable in her speech and behaviour, talking very fast. They had been suspicious of Suzie in the past, as she was best friends with another kitchen staff member who did get fired for turning up to work under the influence of drink and drugs, and they used to spend a lot of time together, and often go missing during their break times, where no one else could see them. There just wasn't enough evidence to bring Suzie up in front of the management, so she received a verbal warning, and was told to be on her best behaviour. All eyes remained on Suzie for the foreseeable future.

Suzie had also been involved in sending highly sexually charged text messages to another carer. The carer already had a wife and child, and his wife eventually found the text messages and kicked him out of their house. A cleaner who used to work up on Franklyn unit actually got fired for sending sexually abusive text messages to a lot of the younger kitchen orderlies, trying to be friendly and helpful, but then developing into more sinister undertones. He was sacked immediately.

It wasn't just the carers either; the head of finance was caught having sex on top of a car bonnet with one of the carers, after an awards ceremony. Unlucky for her she was spotted, and the event spread through the home within seconds the next day. They relished the new gossip and it was the hot topic within the smoking shelter. She rather sheepishly had to be spoken to by the owner, and had kept a low profile ever since. The carer recently got awarded the senior carer position. Just like every other industry, sex was everywhere; nursing homes are no different. In a highly stressful environment such as this, emotions and sexual tension run at their highest levels.

Sharon looked gleefully at the hot trolley in front of her.

'Right, let's get this show on the road.'

Sharon begins crashing pots and pans about. She gets out very large silver containers of feed meals and puddings. Feed meals are pureed foods for the residents that couldn't eat solids any more as they were at risk of choking. They would often comprise of very dark and unappetising colours, or very bright and luminous colours. Nothing had changed here from working in the hospitals.

After the feeds were the 'softs'. This meant any food that was able to be mashed with a spoon or fork, for residents who could manage most foods, just not anything that was too tough or required lots of chewing.

Sharon spoons out large dollops of feed mixture and hands it out to Katie and Jenny. Paul comes bounding into the lounge area.

'Right girls, who needs feeding?'

The carers liked the nurses to help feed every lunch and teatime. Even if they were fully staffed, it helped build respect if you as a nurse were seen 'on the floor' and helping out. Even if this meant just helping to feed one resident, it would go in your favour. Of course this wouldn't always be possible. Nursing is a very variable job, and sometimes you simply wouldn't have enough time to do everything, and you had to prioritise your jobs.

'Right, if you can go feed Andrew please Paul, and Jack, if you can go feed little Lucy for me.'

'Okay.'

Sharon hands me a very small bowlful of colourful mixture, dark brown, light cream, and bright orange, with a small spoon. I walk over to Lucy, who is tapping her little feet away to an imaginary rhythm in her head. Her eyes are open and she is looking up at the ceiling. Her right eye has poorer sight than her left, and it seemed variable when you would get an answer from her. Sometimes she would be vocal at random points throughout the day, other times she would keep quiet almost all the time. It was also variable how she would eat, sometimes keeping her mouth firmly shut, and other times opening it rhythmically.

Lucy was ninety five. She had two sons and a daughter. There was a rift between the sons and daughter when Lucy was starting to get quite ill. The sons blamed the daughter for not getting Lucy into care sooner and were worried that her rapid deterioration was caused because she was not able to be introduced to an efficient medication regime sooner. The daughter was in denial and refused to believe her mother was ill, but merely just getting older. The sons described times when their mother would ring them up at random intervals during the night and ask them if they were coming round to tea. These were the big warning signs to the sons, and they fought to get her into care as soon as possible, whilst the daughter got angry with the sons and kept telling them that their mother was just old and forgetful.

You would have to phone the sons, and then ring the daughter separately, as they wouldn't communicate between each other. Family dynamics played an important and pivotal role in mental health, but it was not up to us to get involved with family conflict. We were here to do a job, and our job was to look after residents and support the family as best we could, not to take sides or get involved in disputes.

I turn to Lucy and look her directly in the eye.

'Hello Lucy.'

A pause.

'Would you like some dinner Lucy, are you hungry?'

'No.'

'Are sure Lucy?'

'No.'

'Would you like a drink instead, Lucy?'

'Yes, all right then!'

There is a drink at the table for Lucy. It has been thickened so that it resembles a very poorly made slush puppy. I try my first spoonful of the orange squash and gently push it up to Lucy's lips.

'Here you are Lucy, I have a drink for you, it's orange.'

The spoon remains by Lucy's lips. Lucy is not moving her lips. Her inquisitive eyes are just staring back at me.

The orange substance is starting to melt a little and drip all down Lucy's chin.

'Lucy.'

I put the spoonful back and tap the spoon a little against the beaker, to try and provide an audio cue. I put the spoonful back up to Lucy's lips. Still nothing. I continue to hold it there for a good few seconds, wondering how I am going to feed Lucy.

I put the spoonful back in the beaker, and place the beaker on the table. All of a sudden Lucy starts moving a little in her seat. She's looking a little uncomfortable, her little arms and hands are trying to push herself up out of the seat and move a little bit. She raises herself a few inches, and then puts herself back down, and while she is momentarily in the air for a few seconds she suddenly shouts out.

'Nnnnnnnnnnnnononononnononnonononononononono.'

She sits back down.

'Lucy are you okay?'

'Yyyyyyyyyyyyyyyyyyyyyyyyyyyyyyyyyyyyyyy...Yes.'

Lucy has the longest stutter I have ever heard. I sat patiently waiting for her to speak the words she wished to say.

'Lucy, are you hungry?'

'Yes.'

I try a spoonful of the rainbow colours of feed meal, and raise the spoon up to Lucy's mouth. As if by magic Lucy suddenly opens her mouth wide and takes the whole spoonful of food in and begins chewing it.

'Is that nice Lucy?'

'Mmm, that's nice, yes.'

I continue to repeat giving Lucy small spoonfuls of her lunch, and it seems to be going well. I had to pause quite often as Lucy wouldn't always open her mouth. Mental health required an unprecedented amount of patience; it was clear to see why it was listed as one of the more stressful jobs you could take on.

The mealtimes would last between half an hour to forty five minutes, depending on the amount of staff at any one time. On average there could be about eight or nine feeds which required a staff member to feed each resident. Some of the soft diets also needed feeding to residents, and then once this was done the rest of the food was dished up and served to residents who could still eat by themselves with normal cutlery.

Once Paul had finished feeding Andrew it was time for him to do the lunchtime medication. Just like the hospitals there were three medication rounds in the daytime, and one bedtime medication round. The morning medication round could take up to an hour and a half, the lunchtime one about forty minutes, teatime about an hour and a half. The bedtime round, about thirty minutes. This was all valuable time, but medication was one of the most important areas of nursing. Get this wrong and you could be in big trouble.

Paul beckons me over.

'Hey Jack, do you want to help me run some drugs to people?'

'Yeah, sure.'

I finish feeding Lucy. She immediately goes back to sleep, but is still tapping her feet on the floor.

I walk over to Paul who is getting out the lunchtime medication on the portable trolley. Everyone's name is contained in a big file, and all their medication is detailed on one big check list for the month; each day has a box to sign for each medication. Most of the medication is already done for you in blister packs, allowing you to pop out the pills into medication pots simply and accurately. You still had to double check everything, as it was very easy to make mistakes by becoming complacent. Paul went through the list and started preparing tablets.

'Okay, can you just take this to Jim, in room seventy one, he doesn't normally take them off me, so see if a new face might help.'

I take a small medicine pot containing a bright yellow tablet and a small round white tablet, and a small pot of water.

I walk around to room seventy one where Jim is sat in his chair with half his lunch on his plate, and half on the floor. His table is a complete mess of sausages and mash. He has white hair combed back straight into a Jack Nicholson type cut, and he stares at me with his big bulging brown eyes.

'Hi Jim, I've just got your tablets for you.'

Jim immediately shouts back at me.

'Well I don't want them any more, so fuck off, I've already had some today.'

I had become hardened to bad language in my student years. It was common, as was refusal of medication.

I remembered back to one of my first instances of being exposed to the bad language that could manifest itself within mental health. It had all happened on my first day, on a dementia ward. I had already been a little shocked and a little emotional as to what I had seen on this ward, through visiting it a few weeks beforehand. Upon my arrival at the ward, I was greeted by a gentleman wearing a green chequered shirt and a waistcoat neatly over it. Wearing thick gold rimmed glasses, the gentleman immediately smiled at me and started to mimic golf swings with his hands.

'Oh you play golf do you?' I asked the gentleman.

He smiled at me, turned to walk in the other direction and stuck his bottom out at me and emitted a high pitched fart, and walked off. There was another gentleman sat down quietly along the corridor. By this point there were a few other nursing assistants stood next to me. The gentleman was looking all three of us up and down.

He smiled at me, and one of the assistants started to speaking to him.

'Hello Derek, how are you ?'

Derek looked at all three of us, his eyes inquisitive. He started speaking. He looked at the first nursing assistant.

'You're a cunt.'

Derek didn't blink an eye. He looked at the other nursing assistant.

'You're a cunt.'

He looked me up and down.

'But you're all right soldier.'

Derek saluted me, and I saluted back and smiled. Welcome to mental health.

I remember many of the shifts as a student nurse where I was trying to give people medication and they would often just spit them out at me or throw them on the floor. It became even worse when you had to try and medicate someone with some Lorazepam to try and calm them down. Often they were in such an agitated state that gently trying to ease a pill into their mouth was the last thing on their mind, and you would often spill the water in the medicine pot down your top or over your hair, and the pills would shoot across the room, sometimes never to be found again.

'Jim, you did have some earlier in the morning.'

'Well that was enough so fuck off.'

'Jim, do you know what these tablets are for?'

'Yes they make you go to the toilet.'

'They're your regular medication that you take each day, they will make you feel better.'

Jims eyes bulged even more, which I didn't think was at all possible.

'Better?! I feel like a pig swimming in shit!!'

I sit on Jim's bed, and gradually move the pot of pills towards him. He immediately hits out at me and knocks the pot of pills flying. The pills go onto the floor.

'I told you I didn't fucking want them, now just listen to me!'

I quickly scoop the pills up from the floor and place them back into the medicine pot.

'Okay Jim, what do you want me to know?'

'I think you need to sit here and have a lecture from me!'

'Okay, what's the lecture about?'

'About these pills, I don't want them any more, so you can tell the man about them, I've had enough!!'

Jim was getting very agitated indeed, his legs were trying to hit out at me, and his fist was raised and rigid, but I was sat just far enough away from his reach if he decided to punch or kick me.

'Okay Jim, I'm going now.'

I wasn't going to push Jim any further; it was his right to refuse his medication, and he was clearly getting very agitated with it. I walked back out to Paul.

'Nope, he's not going to take them,' I say regretfully.

'Didn't think so, he does get quite paranoid and suspicious at times, but sometimes a new face helps. Ah well, I'll mark that down.'

You could always mark a refusal of medication down. It was difficult at times, and some days not everyone was going to be so amenable to taking pills. This was just one of the uphill struggles that you could face on a daily basis.

I could hear Mindy shouting out in the lounge area to the carers.

'Can I go to the toilet please?'

'Of course you can!' Sharon points towards the corridor.

Mindy would often ask each and every lunchtime if she could go to the toilet. Sometimes she would call Paul 'Miss'; it seemed she thought she was still at school at times. She started walking towards Paul and I. She didn't like to walk past the corridor where we were as there were two large windows either side, and as we were on the second floor you could see down to the garden area below. Mindy didn't like any kind of heights and got a bit of vertigo just walking past and she would often outstretch a hand to anyone who was near to the window to help her walk across. She caught my eye and shouted.

'Jack! Come and take me will you.'

She outstretched her hand to me, and I grabbed it, and walked her along the few short steps past the large windows.

'Right, thank you...I'm just going to the toilet okay?!'

I nod in agreement, and Mindy makes her way around the corner to the toilet. Mindy would often shout very loudly when she was asking people to do things for her. She had also seemed to lose any sense of tact or manners. I could see Mindy being the type of lady right at home in a bingo hall in Blackpool, later out for fish and chips from the local chippy. She was down to earth and didn't care what people thought of her.

Paul started preparing some more tablets, quickly popping them out of the relevant blister packs. He poured a small amount of Lactulose out into one of the small medicine pots. Lactulose helped to soften your stools, and helped promote good bowel movements. I remember in the hospital that they used to have litres of the stuff. It tasted like pure treacle and sugar, and it got everywhere, it was incredibly sticky. It was used a lot with elderly care.

'Right okay, this one is for Daniel, just round the corner. I think he is sat in his chair at the minute, room 64, you can't miss him.'

I grab the medicine pot off Paul and walk swiftly to Daniel's room. The room is different from the others in the fact that it has laminated flooring rather than a carpet. I notice there is a rather tall man sat in a recliner, out of initial view from me.

I walk around to the front of the recliner, where I could see Daniel. I had already checked his picture from his notes, so I was sure it was him. Daniel had a number of scars on his face, from numerous falls around the unit. He had a very egg shaped head, and barely a whisp of a hair on it. It was cut short to at least a number one grade. He had dark menacing brown eyes and a very pointed nose. He looked quite mean looking and you certainly wouldn't want to mess with him in a darkened alley. He was just staring out of the window, he barely looked at me as I walked in. He was very thin, and from his position in his chair, it was quite apparent that he was quite tall in stature. I introduced myself to him.

Nothing. Not a smile, not a raise of an eyebrow. Daniel kept staring out of the window.

'Daniel, I have your tablet for you.'

He briefly glances up at me, and I slowly move the plastic medicine spoon towards his mouth. He immediately opens it, and starts crunching down on the tablets. I then place the medicine pot full of Lactulose towards his lips. He purses them together and takes a few sips of the liquid. I wait a few moments and let him swallow, then try to push the last of it towards his lips.

Daniel suddenly fires up into action, like an electric shock had jolted him awake.

'Go away will you, that's enough.'

I retract the medicine pot from his lips. I wait a few moments, then try again.

'That's enough, fuck off will you!!'

I wait a few more moments, then try again.

'Nooooooo I said.'

I wasn't going to try any more. I had given it enough attempts, and he had most of the liquid and tablets off me. Most tablets can be given in dispersible form, either dissolved in liquid, or tablets that will dissolve instantly on the tongue. These were often a lot costlier than normal tablets. If it was up to me I would put everyone on as much dispersible medication as possible. You often found that with the elderly, they would crush and chew on tablets rather than swallow them as they often did not understand what they were being given. This could sometimes affect the efficacy of the tablets, as some were designed to be dissolved gradually over time in the stomach.

I watched Daniel crush and chew the last of his remaining tablets. He looked up at me, then out of the window again. I was just about to leave when Daniel started coughing. It started out a very small cough, but then started to progress to very severe coughing, and gasping of breath. I panicked, and shouted out for Paul.

'Paul!'

Luckily Paul was only just around the corner, and came rushing to my rescue. Daniel was coughing much more frequently now, but would occasionally be gasping for air, and getting more and more panic stricken in his eyes, as though he was trying to clear something in his throat but couldn't quite grasp what was going on. The sounds were very loud coming out from his throat, making a rattly whining sound every time he gasped for air.

Paul immediately leant him forward. He drew his hand back and started to give Daniel big hard smacks to his back, in between his shoulder blades.

Thwack.

Daniel coughed a little, still gasping for air.

Thwack.

Daniel's eyes were bulging, and he continued to cough a little, but was still gasping for air, his face going bright red.

Thwack.

Daniel stopped breathing for a second. A faint swallowing noise could be heard.

'That's it Daniel, swallow it' Paul shouted.

Thwack.

Daniel swallowed again. Everything went silent. You could hear a pin drop. A thick swallowing sound emanated from Daniel's throat.

'Did that get it Daniel?' Paul shouted out.

Another pause. Daniel opened his mouth.

'Ermmmm yes, yes.'

'Thank god for that' Paul said. Paul wiped his brow, and pushed Daniel back into his seat.

'He can sometimes have these coughing fits. It hasn't happened for months though; we think he is just not realising when to swallow at the right time. You didn't do anything wrong, don't worry, his family have been in touch about it, but there's nothing we can do, it's just the deterioration of his illness.'

'Oh, okay' I sigh, relieved. I looked back at Daniel. He was now staring at both Paul and I. I wondered what was going on in his head at this moment in time. He looked a little puzzled. I leave the room with Paul. Paul had almost finished the medication. I was glad he had; it hadn't been the most successful of medication rounds so far. But this was to be expected; it really was such a variable working environment, you never knew what would be round the corner.

I follow Paul round to the nursing office and sit down. Paul is going through his emails.

'Busy day so far eh?!' Paul says.

'Yeah, sure is.'

'Have you had any busier in your training? I bet you have seen some sights.'

I thought carefully for a moment; I had indeed seen some sights. I told Paul about one of the more bizarre sights I had seen at the start of my second year. I was working in a private acute hospital for younger males. Mainly cases of psychosis and schizophrenia. I had only been there a few days and was trying to get to know the residents there, and was getting on quite well with an Indian chap named Naji. He was in his early twenties, often hearing voices that troubled him. I was sat with him in the rather deluxe looking lounge area and chatted to him about his general interests and hobbies. He suddenly looked a little worried.

'I need you to help me with something.'

'Okay, what do you need help with?'

'Well I've been seeing ghosts in my bedroom, and I don't know what to do about it, I'm scared and worried.'

'I doubt there are ghosts in there.'

'Well who do you think I should call?'

I couldn't resist such an easy set up, and just went with it without thinking.

'The Ghostbusters?'

'No I don't think they will help, I need you to come and check with me to see that there's nothing there.'

Naji persisted for quite some time about the ghosts in his room, so much so that I agreed to go and help him look. I had only met him a few times, so I was immediately cautious. My training had taught me to always be aware of where the exits were, and never back yourself into a corner with a patient that you are not familiar with, or even one you are familiar with.

I walked cautiously behind Naji, and had a peek at his room from the corridor.

'Nope, can't see anything at all, I think you're safe.'

Naji still looked rather worried, and kept ushering me to step in further into his room. I ventured a few gentle steps into his room, but I was still only a moment away from the exit and ready to leave quickly if I needed to.

'Nope, still can't see any Naji, I think you're safe, let's go back into the lounge shall we?'

Naji disappeared quickly behind his wardrobe, and I could hear a loud clanking noise, like the sound of metal hitting metal. It was moments later that I realised what I was actually hearing was the sound of Naji taking off his belt, and dropping his trousers.

Naji suddenly reappeared from around his wardrobe, only this time he was crouched on his knees, his trousers and pants fully removed, and he was masturbating furiously in front of me, ushering me to come closer.

I immediately panicked, and rushed out of the room.

'No Naji, I don't want to see that thank you!'

I rushed straight back up the corridor and found the nearest nurse I could; luckily there was a nurse coming down the other way.

'Naji, ermm, Naji is, well, ermm...'

I hadn't really thought about how to phrase the terminology.

'Well, he's ermm, playing with himself!'

The nurse smiled.

'Ah yes, he can do that quite often, he likes the young males I'm afraid, go and tell the manager in the office and document it in the nursing notes.' And with that the nurse carried on walking down the corridor grinning to himself.

Paul smiled at me, and shook his head.

'You get to see it all in mental health eventually, that's all I'm going to say.' Paul continued to smile.

'Oh, I've got an email from Jennifer here, they have signed you up for some venepuncture training, and you need to read this and print something out.'

'Really? Okay then.'

Venepuncture training, taking bloods, was something that I was not particularly keen on, but I guessed that it would look good for the CV. Paul lets me read the email over his shoulder. It requires a bit of a quiz first, and for me to print off some documentation. I decide it would be best to go and do the quiz at home, so I figure it will be a good idea to go down and get some paper so I can print off the relevant details at home. I excuse myself from the office and make my way down to the reception area. I walk past the cheerful lady on reception, and towards the photocopier. I can see Jennifer already there staring at the photocopier in disbelief with another burly looking man who is shaking his head at it.

'Looks like I'll need to order a new part for it.' The burly man continues to shake his head.

'Right, well we need this fixed as soon as possible!' Jennifer barks her orders at the burly man, and he goes scuttling off into another corridor. I can see where the paper tray is to the photocopier and gently brush past Jennifer and open the tray in order to get some paper.

'Hi Jack, what can I do for you?' Jennifer barks at me.

'Hi, I've just read the email you sent Paul, and I just need to get some paper so I can print some stuff out back at home for the Venepuncture training you have put me on.'

'Paper?'

'Yes, I need some paper so I can print this out at home, because there is a quiz involved before I can go to the training.'

'Well why haven't you got any paper at home?'

'Well, normally I have but in this instance I have run out of paper at home, and I notice that the training is only next week, so I thought this would save me a lot of time.'

'How many pieces of paper do you need?'

'Not sure, only about 15-20 sheets?'

'15-20 Sheets! Well if we gave the next ten people that much, that's about 150 pieces of paper!'

'Well, yes, but it's just me asking for it.'

'Listen, the company is not responsible for supplying you with paper for training, that's your own responsibility I'm afraid, I can't condone that.'

I felt my blood beginning to boil.

'Well, I'm not stealing the paper, it is for a legitimate reason, it's for training that you put me on!'

'That may well be, but the company's position is final; we are not providing you with paper, you will have to get your own I'm sorry.'

'So I can't have any paper for training you want to send me on ?'

'No, the company's decision is final, I'm sorry but we're not a charity here.'

'Okay, fine.'

I didn't wish to lose my job so soon in my career, so I just dropped the issue. I couldn't believe it. I walked back past the reception area and up the stairs, back onto the unit.

I walked straight back into the nursing office and told Paul exactly what had happened. He shook his head and laughed.

'I don't believe it mate, I really don't, you do have to watch that Jennifer, she can be an absolute tyrant at times. It doesn't surprise me though, I'd tell them to stick their training right up their arse if I were you, but I know you want the job, so I understand.'

It was true I didn't really want to be taking people's bloods. I just couldn't believe Jennifer's attitude towards me on something so trivial; if they wanted to keep their staff and improve morale, this certainly didn't seem the way to do it. This was supposed to be a flagship home, and if this is the way they treated people no wonder people were so low in mood and had lost all enthusiasm for the role. Maybe this is how they remained so profitable and won so many awards. I wasn't sure how much paper cost these days. Obviously too much to spare me a few pieces.

The company's position was 'final', this was the phrase to remember.

Training was a continual requirement. Many mandatory training sessions happened each year: manual handling, food hygiene, fire safety, etc., etc. Half the staff hadn't done all their training, but the home was intent on getting everyone up to scratch and fully trained up on everything they needed. The home usually notified staff of training courses by letter. They appeared a little threatening in their nature as they would often state that 'failure to attend will result in a charge of £50', just to ensure full attendance.

It was coming up to 12:45 p.m., and most of the lunch had been served up, and all the residents were busy eating the last of their puddings.

Emma comes walking into the office area. She looks a little concerned.

'Paul, can I have a quick word with you?'

'Yeah sure Emma, what's up?'

'It's about Laura. I've got concerns again over her feeding the residents. I was working with her yesterday, and it's not getting any better.'

Paul looks like he has heard this story before, and lets out a little groan.

'Okay, go on.'

'I just don't think she is feeding them properly. She's not being patient enough with them. People like Daniel and Bob always eat their food; she is coming back within a few minutes saying that they only ate half their lunch or breakfast. This has been going on a while now and I'm concerned. I have already spoke to Jennifer about the matter, and she has just brushed me off, saying that she will look into it, but without any hard evidence there's nothing she can do about it.'

'Okay, well what would you like me to do about it?' Paul says, a little disgruntled.

'Well, I think this needs raising again with Jodie.'

Jodie was the unit manager.

'I know Jodie has already spoken to her once, and I think we need to give her a bit more time you know.'

'Well, I'm telling you now Paul, I don't feel comfortable with the way she is acting, and if this goes on any further I am going to take this higher, because I feel that no one is listening to me, and it's the residents that are suffering. I am just not happy with her, it's too soon for her to have come back.'

'Okay, I appreciate where your coming from, I will mention it again to Jodie, and keep an eye, it will be listened to I promise.'

Emma looks at Paul, then at me, and walks off in a sprightly manner.

Paul turns to me.

'And the hits just keep on hitting.'

Laura had been living with her husband for about ten years, seemingly with no problems, until it all started to falter a little within the last year. Laura was approaching her mid forties and had become increasingly tired of her job within the home. She was often seen at the local pub most daytimes drinking alone. Initially she used to drink with her husband, but they had become more argumentative towards each other due to her often erratic work pattern and hours, but Laura had continued to frequent the local pub to drown her sorrows and the stresses of the job. Paul had seen her in there a few times himself, as he liked the odd drink, but only on social occasions. Laura had started to become a little too familiar with the pub, and it had started to escalate so much so that it had interfered with her work.

One morning when Laura was due to start a shift, she had come, as normal, and on time. About forty five minutes into the shift, staff members had started to smell alcohol on her. They raised their concerns to the nurse in charge, and they ordered an inspection of Laura's bag. Within the bag was a bottle of Lucozade. Upon further inspection of the bottle, it was revealed that the bottle of Lucozade contained vodka.

Laura was immediately sent home that day, and ordered to clean up her act. Many interventions from the management ensued, and even Jennifer had visited Laura at her home on a number of occasions to provide support and help for Laura. Laura was finally ready to come back to work, initially on a reduced number of hours. It had worked well for a number of weeks, but now the carers were starting to complain. They felt that Laura wasn't doing her job properly, and was starting to jeopardise the safety and well being of the residents. Management had taken a blind eye approach to the problem so far, and tried to give Laura the benefit of the doubt, and she had been spoken to since coming back, and asked if she thought that she was taking on too many hours. She stated that she was able to cope with the stresses of the job just fine, and had been managing not to drink for a number of weeks. The carers were not so sure, and the complaints had been starting to rise.

It would carry on for many more months. She would turn up to work smelling strongly of alcohol, but nothing would be done. One morning the manager of the unit noticed Laura smelt strongly of alcohol. She went to see the manager of the home about it, but Laura wasn't sent home. The unit was very short staffed, so the manager just let Laura continue to work her shift and kept a close eye on her. This would open the eyes of the other employees considering doing the same, sending a message throughout the company that if it was okay for one, then it could be okay for many to engage in illicit behaviour, and still keep their job.

Paul turned to me.

'This is the hardest part of the job, keeping the carers happy. Between that and the relatives, you barely have time for the residents some days!'

I heeded Paul's advice with caution.

'They don't miss a trick these carers; if they don't like something they will tell you, mark my words. I try to appease everyone, but it just isn't possible all the time I'm afraid, but you can only do your best can't you? I think I'm just too damn nice at times, and nice guys finish last.'

'It certainly seems a challenge!'

'The knives are out for Laura, and they take no prisoners here, they'll hang her for this, you mark my words.'

> *'My father taught me many things here — he taught me in this room. He taught me — keep your friends close but your enemies closer.'*

<u>Michael Corleone</u> in <u>The Godfather Part II</u> (1974)

1–2 p.m.

Paul slams the office phone down.

'I don't believe this!'

'What's up?' I say.

'I've got to cover Gerald unit for an hour. One of their nurses has gone off sick and they can't find cover until an hour's time when another nurse can come in.'

'Okay.'

'Sorry mate, I'm going to have to leave you in charge for an hour. The carers will look after you though, and this is a quiet time of the day. I'm really sorry to have to do this to you, I have no choice, Jennifer has told me'

'Erm, okay.'

Paul hands me the huge bunch of keys, and advises me just to stay calm and ask the carers if I need anything. And with that Paul was off down the corridor to the other unit. I sat in the office area for a moment, just wondering how the hell I was going to cope with everything.

Jenny comes up to me and offers me a drink. I gratefully accept. The phone suddenly rings.

I answer the phone hurriedly.

'Hello, Jack speaking.'

The phone system was supposed to protect each unit from getting hundreds of calls each day; any phone call would come through to the reception area first and then be diverted accordingly to the unit it was destined for. I could tell it wasn't an outside line because the phone simply said 'guest' on the LCD display. This was probably from reception.

'Hi, I have Dwayne's wife on the line for you.'

'Err ok, yes,' I stumble out.

'Just putting you through.'

The phone clicks off, and then silence. There is a faint whisper of a voice on the other end of the phone line.

'Hello there, I'm just wondering how Dwayne has been today please.'

I had remembered going in to feed Dwayne this morning, and I had the handover notes in front of me to tell his wife how he had been during the night. I found it was often helpful to be prepared when talking to residents' relatives. Luckily here, as opposed to the hospital, the handover notes were typed up each day and night so there was an ongoing record of any changes in the residents' behaviour, also any changes from the weekly ward rounds were indicated next to each resident's name, a far more efficient way of documenting and one that I found a lot easier, as you would often try to scrabble for information on a resident, and this just made it a lot easier as it was written down.

'Hi, he was a little agitated this morning when we were giving him his breakfast, but appears to have settled a bit now, the night staff reported a good night's sleep.'

'Oh okay, that's brilliant thank you very much, goodbye.'

I put the phone down. Relatives could vary from my experiences in the hospital and what Paul had filled me in on:

The 'ringers' - Some relatives would ring up every day, just a quick phone call to check on how their relatives were doing. They would usually ring at precisely the most inconvenient times, either first thing in the morning, when you were doing the morning medication, or last thing in the evening, just as you were finishing off your tea time medication. They wouldn't keep you for very long, and all they would require was a few bits of minor information.

The 'dailies' - Others would visit every day. Every single day, without fail, usually at a specific time, around mealtimes, so they could help their relative with their meal. You could set your watch by the daily visitors. The daily visitors could be a massive bonus to the working day, as they were an extra pair of hands, helping free up the carers to help other residents with their food.

The 'no shows' - Relatives who hardly visited at all, as they found it far too painful to see their wife or husband with their illness. Some relatives were either too far away to travel, or simply didn't wish to make the effort to visit. You might see these relatives once a year if you were lucky, either on a birthday or another holiday occasion such as Christmas. They often wouldn't bother the nursing staff at all. They would simply come in and spend a few moments with their significant others, and then quietly leave.

The 'nightmares' - Relatives from hell. Relatives that thought they knew absolutely everything about their father or mother's illness and would try to tell you how to do your job. These relatives would ring, as well as visit, almost daily, and would require continual updates, phoning for minor changes in their mum or dad's behaviour. If a resident was prone to a lot of falls, then they would require you to ring them every time they fell. You had to be sure you documented absolutely every change in presentation. You would frequently spend more time looking after the relative rather than the resident at times.

Often they would try to suggest medication that they thought was needed, and considerable pressure would be put on the nursing team to appease them. If they didn't like how you were doing things, they would have no problems at all speaking to the doctor directly or complaining directly to the owner of the home. These people kept you on your toes.

The 'worried well' – These were the relatives that worried about absolutely everything, from a tiny scratch on their husband's foot, to them not taking their normal cup of squash in the afternoon. They spotted everything, and would come to the nursing team about everything. They required a lot of reassurance and time, something that wasn't always in great abundance. I'm not sure if they trusted the nursing staff or not, or merely just wanted to keep a check on what we were doing, but they would ask hundreds of questions in any given day about the most minor of areas, but you had to pay attention, and if you didn't action what they wanted, they would simply go and ask all the other nurses about it as well.

Is nursing a thankless task?

After a year of working as a qualified nurse, managing a unit on my own, I had a phone call from a relative. It was right at the end of my shift, and made me question sometimes how nursing can sometimes seem quite a thankless task.

I documented and emailed my manager at the time on exactly what the relative had discussed with me and his attitude towards me. I had had no previous problems with the relative, and he had shown no previous malice or disgruntled feelings towards me. Here is the full transcript of the email, and just goes to show exactly how hard it can be sometimes to appease everyone as a qualified nurse:

Hi Jennifer,

I just need to email you about a phone call I have just had regarding Mr X (Mrs X's husband).

A few points he raised:

- He was unhappy about not being able to get through to the unit today in particular, saying he had tried four times this evening. When he eventually did get through he made quite an accusatory attack on the fact that myself and Y didn't appear to answer the phone very often when we were on shift (not just this shift, but other shifts as well).
- He complained that I did not greet him today, even though I'm sure I did (however I was off the unit for an hour, whilst he was visiting. He visited between 2pm – 3pm. I was off the floor from 2.03pm – 2.53pm as I took my morning break which I didn't have the chance to have

due to having podiatry training and my lunch break all in one go). He stated that he observed us both to be just 'flicking paper' in the office today, and particular commented on the fact that when I returned back to the unit after my break I did not greet him, and simply wondered straight into the office and 'turned paper'. He asked me how I could know what was going on in the unit by walking back into the office. I explained that Y was also on duty today, and Y had coincidentally just spent a lot of time talking to Mr X himself. I explained that Y would immediately have notified me of any changes to any residents, and she was well aware when I was due back on the unit as I always notify where I am and how long I will be.

- He complained he didn't realise who was in charge today, and that there was not enough communication on the unit.
- Not being formally introduced to our new carer and any of the other new carers, and did not understand how 'domestics' could suddenly become carers. He was making complaints about how he didn't see how they could become a carer so quickly, despite me explaining to him that these carers had both had extensive experience of being a carer in other establishments previously.
- He complained that when he first arrived on this unit, he was never shown how to access the garden area.
- He complained about general communication within the home in general, complaining that he had researched many other homes in the area before picking the home, and commented on the fact that the home had 'won so many awards' but what he was seeing seemed to paint a different picture, and he was very concerned

and worried about not being able to get through.
- He was concerned about Mrs X having slept for most of the time of his visit today (about an hour). Mrs X has recently had her Matrifen patch increased to 25mcg (from 12mcg) and has had a recent decrease in her Aricept. Mrs X had a tendency to wander this morning, and later ate all her tea and continued to wander throughout the afternoon and evening.
- He stated that in his working day he used to manage over 40 people, and knows all about handling people and communication and implied that things needed to improve.
- He complained that when he first took Mrs X to the home, he was not introduced formally to the manager, and only realised later after the event.
- He also complained about last Saturday being particular difficult to get through on the phone (I believe this was a shift when Y was in charge but incredibly short staffed).
- He complained that he observed me to be doing my nursing notes in the lounge area, and stated why couldn't I be doing them in the office (so I would be free to answer the phone!) I stated that I often did my notes in the lounge area so I could keep an eye on the residents, as there were a lot of residents who were at risk of falling, and this has been agreed as a sensible thing to do by Jodie in a recent nursing meeting, so we can keep the lounge area observed as best we can, and always go to the phone when we can hear it ringing.
- He stated he heard the phone ringing a number of times this afternoon and that Y and other members of staff were not seen to be answering it (whilst I was off the unit) despite me explaining to him that there are two distinct ring tones that will identify the phone for main reception or unit.

This phone call happened at approximately 7:30 p.m. this evening, and lasted a good half an hour. During this time, I felt the focus shifted from not just a personal attack on myself and Y, but also the home in general, saying that it 'wasn't just him' that was worried, and about other relatives, and what if they wanted to get through?

I felt I had to personally defend my nursing actions, and on numerous times explained to him that whilst I did my best to answer the phone as best I could, there were key times when it may not always be convenient to do so, most notably in the morning time during the morning medication. Mr X will often ring around 9 a.m. to ask how Mrs X is, and I often do speak to him. I explained that when he may not be able to get through, this might mean that the nurses in charge are doing the medication round, morning or tea. I personally do not tend to answer the phone whilst doing a medication round.

I personally feel that I will get easily distracted and make mistakes. In the past when first working here, I felt a slight pressure to continue to answer the phone whilst doing a medication round. I personally feel that this is unsafe practice, and at the end of the day, I do not want to get disciplined for making a drug error, which I feel would easily happen one day; if you are answering the phone continually, it is very easy to break concentration. Other nurses may be able to do this, but I do not feel comfortable with this, or feel I should be put under this sort of pressure. I prioritise the medication rounds as being of the utmost importance during the day, and continually check and recheck to make sure there is no room for error. I do not wish to lose my registration over such an error.

> I also explained that whilst I personally do make efforts to answer the phone, a dementia unit is incredibly variable, and any manner of things can happen in a split second, as I am sure you are aware; people getting agitated, falling over, and requiring immediate attention. He said he appreciated this, but his tone and manner still seemed to me a personal attack. I am well aware of the strains both mentally and emotionally on relatives of people with dementia. I feel I have an excellent working relationship with most of the relatives here, and I am sure that if you asked them they would agree. I always try to go out of my way to be kind and civilised and speak to them whilst still doing my nursing duties. This really has made feel like nursing is a very thankless task at times.
>
> I feel that it is very important for you to be updated on this. I asked Mr X if he had these concerns would he like to pass them on further, but he declined. He ended the phone call quite abruptly.
>
> If Mr X wants to make a formal complaint about me or Y, then he can, but I think I would be justified in making a complaint back to him, as I do not think as nurses we should put up with this kind of talk, bordering on the abusive, and telling us how to do our jobs. If you think his complaints are valid, then please do tell me. But I don't think it is fair to be treated this way.
> Jack
>
> Jennifer never replied or discussed this matter with me despite this exhaustive email.

In the hospital I remember the nurses saying to me that the hardest part of the job was dealing with the families. It was a difficult one to call; a lot of the relatives here seemed very nice, but you always had to be aware that if there was one thing that they didn't like about their relative's care, then they would soon tell you.

Jenny placed down a fresh hot cup of coffee down by me.

'There you go, how are you getting on then ?'

'Yeah, not too bad, getting there slowly, it's been a busy day so far.'

'Yep, and it will probably get busier.'

Jenny had a heart of gold, and she worked hard. She didn't really need the money, so it was clear that she was doing it for the love of the job, despite all the rules and regulations and stresses that would get everyone down. She had been in the business of care for fifteen years, and she was hopefully going to wind down her hours gradually over the next few years and maybe move abroad with her husband. Good quality carers were often hard to come by, and usually the hospital system spat them out at a terrific rate, leaving them deflated and depressed about their work, and finding it hard to enthuse about why it was they went into care work in the first place, to look after people. To be caring.

'You going to get some lunch in a bit?'

'Well, Paul's not here and I have the keys for an hour.'

'Oh don't worry, if you go to the staff room, we can always get hold of you, it's not far, everything is fine here and I will let you know if anything needs doing; you're only a door away'

'I should stay on the unit really.'

'Okay, well why don't you have a sandwich in the quiet lounge? No one will bother you there anyway.'

'Okay, will do.'

I grab my bag from the office and unpack my lunch in the quiet lounge. I can hear the hustle and bustle of the unit and the last clanking of the lunch cutlery. Around this time, the residents would be toileted. Not all residents, just the ones that were not able to attend to their own personal hygiene needs. This was often a fairly quick process, and Sharon and Katie were bustling past the lounge area with residents in wheelchairs, with Emma following.

This was the first true break of the day, and I was shattered. At least the time went quickly. I used to remember many of the jobs I used to do before becoming a nurse, and how the time seemed to last forever. My feet hadn't touched the ground since starting here.

My initial anxieties had settled a little, but the pace of the unit had seemed so quick, particularly this morning. I guessed it would get better, and I had to think that I wouldn't always be on the floor so much as I would have my nursing duties to attend to.

I look at the fish in the fish tank in the far corner. They looked so peaceful. I could feel my stress levels building a little, but tried my best to keep them down.

Suddenly Emma came bolting around the corner and into the quiet lounge.

'Jack! Can you come quickly, Vancy has fallen over.'

My heart sank. I quickly rushed up the corridor, to where Vancy was. She was sat in Jim's room next to a chair, with her forehead bleeding. She was still garbling some incoherent speech to herself, appearing oblivious to what had happened. She had obviously fallen and the chair had broken her fall slowly. Luckily Paul had told me where the dressing and supplies were kept, so I raced down to the store where they were kept, and desperately tried to find the right key to open the door. Once the door was opened, I stared at everything in front of me, not realising what on earth anything was for.

During your mental health training you really didn't have any training on dressings or wounds. I vaguely remember in the distant past maybe one lecture on wound care, but all I really remember from it is getting into a right mess trying to bandage some of my fellow students up in a sling, and being thrown a book on first aid, and basically being told to 'get on with it'. You certainly were not a real 'adult nurse', and this was becoming a lot more clearer to me as I stared at the wealth of dressings and clear tubes of liquid in front of me.

I had no idea what I was going to do, and then I saw a box of Steri Strips. I remembered these from university, and the hospital. These were just very small strips of sticky tape that helped bring a wound together and hold it in place. I also spied some Irripod saline solution, and some cotton wool balls. I think I was prepared; I tried to breathe slowly and calm myself down. It couldn't be that hard, could it? I would just clean the area with the solution and some cotton wool balls, then patch the wound up with a few strips; simple. I was a nurse.

I closed up the cupboard, and rushed back down to where Vancy was. She was still in the exact same position, and still muttering away to herself.

'I'm frightened, please help me, I'm hurting, I'm hurting, I'm hurting, please please please, I'm hurting, I'm hurting.'

This shouting had started to annoy Jim who was just staring at her in disbelief.

'Tell her to get out of here, she's in my room you know.'

'I know Jim, I will be as quick as possible I promise!'

'You had better be!'

Jim's eyes remained bulging, to the point where they seemed they might well pop out all together. He later settled, and started to play with his table in front of him. Eventually he managed to grab the table with enough force and throw it down onto the floor in front of him. It made a huge banging sound, but after this he seemed to be more relaxed, and gradually started to shut his eyes, with his hands still in mid air, making little fists.

I kneel down to attend to Vancy. I had everything I needed. I gently open the Irripod solution, in a nice easy to use twist off plastic top, which then allows you to gently spray some of the fluid. I nervously spray the fluid onto the cotton wool ball and begin daubing at the wound on Vancy's forehead. It's not a large cut luckily, but there is still enough blood to make me a little queasy, and I realise again why I never trained to become a general nurse. Vancy is still shouting out at the top of her voice, becoming more and more shaky as she continues. I gently wipe up as much of the blood as possible and then apply a few of the Steri Strips. They seem to hold everything together.

Emma and I gradually help Vancy to her feet, and sit her in the chair that moments ago she hit with her head. She immediately tries to push off out of the seat, and stands up straight, and begins walking down the corridor again almost immediately. There was no way to stop her, she was on a mission.

I wander back to the nursing office, and begin going through some of the notes of the residents. The notes were not as detailed as when I worked in the hospital. In the hospital you had files the size of the Bible detailing every single communication between doctors or community teams, in depth medical history, nutritional status, and many more detailed snippets of information that really gave you a good sense of the patient. The notes I was looking through were practically anorexic in comparison. A few sheets of paper with a few minor details about their medical history, and the main bulk of the notes were just pages and pages of daily entries. There wasn't much else to go on, no real history of where they had come from and what mental health teams they may have been involved with before coming to the home.

As I was pouring over the notes in the office, I started to feel a creeping presence standing over me. I look up, and there in the doorway was a slightly scruffy man, who must have been well over six foot tall, towering over me. He was wearing dark blue trousers, and a plain black t-shirt. I could see a name badge faintly above his left breast, which identified him as 'Neil Vice, computer maintenance'. He had short brown spiky hair, and was in his mid forties, with a few days' worth of designer stubble. He smiled at me, and introduced himself.

'Hi mate, Neil Vice, computer technician. I've been asked to upgrade your computer, as it's running slow.'

'You have?'

'Yep, won't take long at all, can you just log off for me, and I'll whip that RAM out of there in no time. We've had some complaints lately, how have you been finding it?'

'Well, I haven't really had much chance with it to be honest, I'm new here today.'

'Aren't you the lucky one! They usually wait around here until all their computers are crawling along, as slow as snails, and then I get a panicky call, saying that a manager cannot get to her emails fast enough, and then I'm sent out. The computers round here are ancient anyway, they just run them into the ground if you ask me, they would rather spend all their money on fancy cars and holidays if you ask me!'

'I can imagine.'

I quickly log off, and Neil Vice reveals a large black bag, full of various bits of wiring, and what appear to be a few computer programming books.

'So your newly qualified then?'

'Yeah, I came straight from university to here!'

'Just keep your head down, and you will be fine. Just watch these walls though, they talk, if you know what I mean.'

'Sure thing.'

Neil quickly removes the back panel off the computer. A few cracking and snapping sounds later, and he comes back from around the computer.

'All sorted mate. Well that's it for me today, I've got a bottle of wine with my name on it at home!'

'Wine? I prefer beer myself.'

'Yeah, I'm bit of a connoisseur...I've probably spilt more wine than you've drunk! Right! Can't hang around here all day, see you around.'

'Yeah, sure.'

Neil Vice packs up his bag and quickly exits the nursing office. Sharon pops her head round into the office.

'Can you ring Mick for us please love, the stand aid isn't working again. Do you know how to do that? His number is on the wall.'

'Err okay, what's wrong with it?'

'The handle just comes off, and the wheel bearing isn't working correctly. We have complained about this before. You need to speak to Mick about it, and hopefully he will come and see it, good luck though.'

Mick was the operations manager, and had overall responsibility for the maintenance and equipment. His nick name from the smoking shelter was 'Mick the prick'. He usually spoke to people rather shortly and sharply, and if he could do anything in his power to save the company any money, he would.

Originally from America, he was best friends with the owner of the company and when he wanted to move back to England the owner sorted him out with a job. Mick would be quite flirtatious with female nurses and carers, using suggestive innuendo and appearing to use his power for his own gains. There had never been any serious allegations, but recently a few of the nurses had started to feel particularly uncomfortable around him, and tried to avoid him at all costs, describing him as slimy and very full of himself.

No one really knew what he actually did. There were many reports from cleaners just observing him to spend large amounts of time walking around the units on his mobile phone talking to his family. Paul would sum his job up as 'jobs for the boys'. Mick was described by Jennifer as a clever man. A clever man who could 'get people out of the company' if he so desired, if they weren't working out as well as they could be. He had ways of knocking employees confidence, arguing with them and wearing them down, little by little.

Jennifer had also been heard to speak to the cleaners in a derogatory way. One of the cleaners had briefly been going out with Jennifer's other daughter. They had split up and consequently the cleaner had been having a hard time of it at work. Jennifer had warned him that she was 'going to make his life hell', and Mick had been complaining every single day to him about dusty corners of rooms and chairs that hadn't been cleaned properly.

'Sure,' I say.

I look up at the wall in front of me. Everyone had extension numbers, and Mick's was detailed there with everyone else's. I picked up the phone and dialled the three digit number. It just kept ringing, then eventually went to answer phone. I leave a quick message for him to contact me at his earliest convenience to look at the stand aid.

The stand aid helped people stand. It was that simple; it was quite a unique device which utilised a material belt that wrapped around the resident under their arms and velcroed them in tightly, then the belt was attached to the machine and allowed you to gradually hoist people up automatically. But due to many hours of constant use, machinery would often break down. It should be used at all times when a resident needs additional assistance to stand. Often it wouldn't get used, and residents would be lifted up with two carers under their arms (known as the drag lift). This would be quicker, but illegal, and more risky if the resident fell or became agitated. The proper equipment was here for our own safety as well as the residents'.

The stand aid was given to the company in the first place, and it had been used well past its sell by date, but the company was very reluctant to spend any sort of money to fix these things if they could get away with it. Paul had said the maintenance man had an ongoing battle with Mick most days about buying light bulbs and very basic items for the home. He would often pull a face if anything cost more than a few pounds. It seems wherever you are in healthcare today, money is always going to be a predominant measure of any success. I had heard horror stories of Mick shouting at nurses and carers and blaming them for any mechanical failure of machines. The stand aid worked by battery, and you needed to charge this battery on a daily basis.

Originally there were two batteries for the stand aid, but no-one knew where the second battery had gone, or had even seen it in the first place. When the staff asked Mick if they could have a second battery, Mick simply said that he couldn't authorise this, and the stand aid battery would simply have to be charged after each and every use. He even uttered the phrase 'It's quite simple isn't it?' In principle this is fine, after each use it can be put on charge, but things would operate a lot smoother and simpler if there was always a spare battery on charge, and if the battery we had happened to malfunction, then there would always be a backup. This just showed you how serious the company was about saving any money they could and making the staff work as hard as they could with the equipment. The stand aid was quite old and even had a very old manual handle system to open its lower legs, which were used to enable smooth flow in and around many of the chairs in the lounge area.

A lot of the cleaners detested Mick. He would frequently not listen to any of them when they tried to voice any opinion. One of the cleaners used a sanitizer machine to completely sanitise a room once a resident had died. According to the sanitizer manual, the various chemicals that the machine would use would actually corrode underlay. Mick refused to believe this, and continued to argue that it didn't, despite it saying it in black and white.

Mick was always right in his mind. Most of the rooms had carpet with underlay, rather than laminate flooring. It was estimated that each room would cost three thousand pounds to laminate, so it would not be cost effective to have every room like this. The carpets were getting worse, and Mick would always blame the cleaners for the state that they were in.

The cleaners were getting 'slaughtered' of late. They didn't have enough supplies or tools to do their job properly. They had been receiving lots of complaints from relatives about the conditions of the rooms. The owner had done a spot check and was not impressed. Mick had not ordered enough of the correct cleaning fluid for one month, and told all the cleaners that they would have to make do with what they had. They had nothing except for washing up liquid. They couldn't even use any scented cleaning products as Mick had refused to order the rest of the cleaning products until the following month.

Some days you were lucky to get a cleaner working on the unit; frequently they would be stretched over the whole home. Some days there wouldn't be a cleaner based in the home at all. Other days they would have to bear the responsibility of all four units, pushed to their absolute breaking point.

I could hear Vancy shouting from around the corner. She was coming towards me into the nursing office.

'Help me please, you sir! Please please help me.'

I usher Vancy into the office and sit her down in the chair next to me, trying to calm her down, but to no avail.

Suddenly the phone rings. It says 'Nurse D' on the LCD display. This means it is from another unit in the building.

'Hello.'

'Hello, Jack is it?'

'Hi, yes it is, can I help?

'Hi, it's Sally, the unit manager from downstairs, can I have a quick word with you? Can you come downstairs and see me.'

'Well, I'm here on my own at the moment and I've got a resident here that has fallen over, so I can't really.'

'Okay love, I'll come up and see you in a minute then.'

'Okay.'

I put the phone down. Paul had warned me about Sally. He had his doubts about her own mental state, and particularly after the Citalopram debacle, he detested her even further. Sally told Paul that once she 'got someone on Citalopram, they stayed on it'. He thought she was potentially manic herself, and had particular suspicions about her being bi-polar. Staff members would often fall foul of her silver edged tongue some days, but other days she would be as nice as pie, very friendly and helping you out in any way she could. Paul would jokingly nickname her the Citalopram kid after that.

Vancy was still shouting out in the office area. I could feel my stress levels rising. I felt hot and sweaty. Deirdre, Mark's wife, appeared at the doorway.

Deirdre was always willing to help as much as she could. She would often do the laundry in the afternoon, and help to wash the medicine pots up as the nurses carried on doing their medication during lunchtime and at teatime. There were never enough medicine pots to satisfy a full medication round. They were plastic, and would continually go missing, but the company would never replace them. You would need at least forty pots at all times, but as they gradually diminished, the nurses were just expected to use what they had left. This would cause a considerable waste of time, especially in the morning, as you were often spending most of your time washing up pots about three or four times during a round. Countless requests had been put forward to either order more medicine pots, or even disposable pots, but to no avail.

The same went with the plastic spoons. In the hospitals, they disposed of the plastic spoons and pots after each round. The same went for the new temperature machine, which required small plastic sleeves, as each sleeve was disposable. Temperature would be taken by placing the machine just inside a resident's ear. The management actually stated that these sleeves would have to be washed each time, rather than disposed of, as it would be too costly to keep purchasing new plastic sleeves. The sleeves would crumple and rip easily; it was not practical or even hygienic to re use these sleeves in this way.

Without Deirdre's help each day, the carers would feel even more pressurised. Deirdre did a fantastic job of keeping the unit going just by helping out with these few simple tasks.

Deirdre was trying to calm Vancy down and offer her some reassurance. I think Deirdre had sensed my stress levels rising and was just trying to offer a hand.

Sally bursts through into the office area. She had blonde curly hair, down to her shoulders, a semi maniacal grin on her face, and wearing an Adidas tracksuit top over her tunic. She points in the general direction of the quiet lounge area. I dutifully follow her in. She shuts the door behind her, and I sit opposite her. She begins in a very low and serious tone as she speaks.

'Now, I know you're new, but I just wanted to have a few words with you about a few things.'

'Okay, sure.'

'Well I get the impression that everyone likes you already, that's not a problem, but I just wanted to make you aware that to really gain respect with the carers for the future you need to be seen on the floor. You are mapping these residents, and you need to be able to see any changes in their behaviour or any physical deterioration.'

'Okay, yeah sure, I realise this, but I am new.'

'Oh, I know. Listen, people have sat me down loads in the past and given me talks, and I have become better for it. Don't think of this as a reflection of your nursing skills, but I am telling you this now so you can start to gain respect from the carers, right from the start.'

'Okay, I understand.'

'Now, it's nothing to do with you. I will be speaking to Paul about the matter too as people have raised issues against him, but because you're new I just wanted to make sure that we were on an even keel, and set you up correctly right from the start.'

'Okay,' I say.

'Care plans are very important, but I would leave all the paperwork till the afternoon, after you have done the morning medication. You need to be out and on that floor getting people up and helping the carers. If they see you on the floor you will gain respect and they will understand that you're not a nurse that just sits in the office.'

Care plans were incredibly important. The care plans had recently been moving towards a more professional and more in depth version. The care plans detail everything about the resident, and provide sufficient information so that if a complete stranger picked up the care plans they would be able to know everything about the resident and their needs. They cover such areas as nutrition, mobility, mental health, diabetes, aggression, etc., etc. You would also have to draw up a care plan if someone had a urine infection, and were being treated for antibiotics, and if ever inspected and spot checked, if these were not up to date, then a home could lose its star status by the commission. It worked a little like hotels: a ranking system. In extreme cases, a home could get shut down if it had poor documentation that was not up to date.

Unfortunately, the work of a nurse was never quite done. What with helping out on the floor as much as possible, it was often incredibly hard to ever complete or get these care plans up to date at all and they would often run several months behind. Paul would often tell me about the various lists that would suddenly appear in the office or in the daily diary about certain areas of the care plans that he was required to complete. Every nurse was assigned four to five residents that they were solely responsible for, in completing their care plans to the highest standard.

A constant battle always ensued between management and the nursing staff. Management wanted all the care plans complete and up to date. Nurses wanted more time to do them. Carers wanted the nurses to be on the floor more helping out, and everyone just generally wanted much more time to do everything.

Care plans would be hand written to a high standard. No one would read them. The only time people would read them was when there was a serious problem. If something had happened with a resident regarding nutritional needs or mobility, then the care plans were the first port of call to investigate to make sure everything was written down in black and white. They could be used as legal documents in any serious pending case against the home or nursing staff.

The move to a more 'relative friendly' and 'patient centred' approach was looming. The management wanted more focus with the care plans; getting the relatives to sign their agreement with everything the nurses had put was going to be rolling out over the next few months.

It had already been trialled with a few units, and the relatives were happy to sign; they trusted the nursing team and were happy to go along with it. Initially they were asked just to sign one piece of paper, but the management wanted to push for more; they wanted relatives to sign every single care plan the nurses wrote. This wasn't always practical. The relatives trusted the nurses for a reason; they were the professionals, and they had every faith in them. Dementia already has a massively emotional impact on a family member, and the last thing they want to be doing is signing lots of paper that remind them about everything.

The nurses eventually had enough, and had argued for some protected time away from the unit in order to do the care plans. This had started to work, but only when there was an ample supply of staff on the unit. And since the suggested requirement of just four staff was the minimum needed to run a unit, this would rarely happen. The care plans just continued to become more and more out of date, despite the best intentions of all nurses. It wasn't just the care plans that often fell behind; the risk assessments were also often out of date, and very rarely updated due to these time constraints.

Whilst I continued to dwell on the importance of these care plans, Sally looked at me, eagerly awaiting my response.

'Okay, yeah sure, but I can see from how Paul works that it's not always going to be that easy. There are relatives to speak to as well, and this unit appears to be a very heavy one.'

'It is, but you're not there for the relatives, you're here for the residents, these are our main concern, and I appreciate that your manager likes to talk and counsel the relatives up here, but that's not what we are here for; it's the residents that matter.'

I pondered over this. Person centred care has its origins in the work of Carl Rogers, and brings together ideas and ways of working with experiences of people with dementia, focusing more on both relationships and communication. Relationship centred care involved a much broader spectrum, involving the families and friends, working together and again placing a strong emphasis on good communication.

To just leave the relatives aside and only focus on the person in our care was actually going against everything I had been taught. I took this advice with a pinch of salt. The notion of relationship extends beyond just three people to other members of the care team. The very nature of dementia affected not just the resident in question but had a huge impact on the families, to a sometimes devastating effect. We couldn't ignore this impact, and we needed to be there for them, as well as looking after their nearest and dearest. They would often need more support than the residents at times, and that in itself could be hugely mentally draining. Sitting with someone with a cup of tea, and talking to them, as they ask you how long their husband has to live. Seeing tears well up in their eyes as you have to tell them that they may only have hours left, and giving them time to grieve.

Whilst I knew the theory, I simply state a meek 'okay', and Sally stands up, and turns one last time to me.

'Is that okay, you don't want to say anything to what I have said do you?'

'No, that's fine,' I lie convincingly.

My blood was already starting to boil. One day I would hope to gain the skills of assertiveness and be bold enough to challenge people's ideas about how they thought things should be. It would be one of my ongoing crusades, and I made a mental note of this. The job was hard enough as it was, without being told that I needed to shift my attitudes and opinions a little, before I had even started. Maybe Paul was right; Sally may indeed have a few issues of her own.

The managers would often have to sit down nurses and carers and have talks with them, if there were ever any concerns or complaints. Whilst the carers should work as a team, it wouldn't always go to plan. Some wouldn't think twice about complaining about their own colleagues. Carers have reported other carers in the past for farting on the unit. Rather than speak to that carer directly, it was taken directly to Jennifer, with a formal letter of complaint. The carer had to come in on her day off and discuss about how unprofessional this was. The carer never found out who had complained about her. In fact they still work closely together on many shifts, with the carer oblivious to the fact that even her closest team mates wouldn't think twice about complaining, even over a small matter.

I remember as a student, I would often think that all nurses used to do was simply sit in the office, but I was already beginning to realise that there was an awful lot of responsibility and work to do that people just wouldn't be able to see going on, but was incredibly important. The amount of paperwork and legal documents that needed to be correctly filled in was a huge undertaking, let alone keeping the relatives updated, and generally keeping the unit running well. It was very easy to pass judgements on people before you knew the true story and what really went on behind the scenes.

Mr Jackson had arrived on the unit to see his wife Maggie. Maggie was relatively new here on the unit and would frequently wander, and was at times tearful. We had to keep a close eye on her as Bob would often try to grab hold of her and not let go. You needed eyes in the back of your head. Mr Jackson was in his mid 60s himself and not too good on his feet either. He often used to sit peacefully in the lounge area whilst his wife bustled around him and walked up and down the corridor. He used to get quite anxious and frustrated that he couldn't sit his wife down for more than a few minutes. He had resigned himself to the fact that his wife wasn't who she used to be, but he came every day without fail, enjoyed a cup of tea with her and then left the unit, saying his goodbyes. He looked like he was hiding a lot of emotional turmoil inside. He hardly ever bothered the nurses with anything. He would ring each morning to check on how Maggie was, and arrive later that afternoon. For him, that's all he could do for Maggie. It was often sad seeing the relatives each day; they were trying their best in dealing with what had happened, and we were here to try and help them in every way we could.

Daniel was slowly making his way towards the nursing office, looking suspicious. It was like watching a secret agent, trying to tiptoe past the office, trying to look as discreet as he possibly could. He was holding on to the hand rails alongside the wall, and shuffling a small amount each footstep.

Paul comes bursting into the office, a thin veil of sweat glistening on his brow.

'Jesus wept! I never want to go on that unit ever again! Next time that happens, I'm throwing them the keys, and saying goodbye!'

'What happened?'

'Where do I start?! For starters a chap was fitting, because his syringe driver wasn't put in properly. They had used the wrong syringe and it had been calibrated all wrong so it wasn't administering the correct dose over the correct amount of time.'

'Wow.'

'Yeah, an absolute nightmare, then there were about a hundred patches to do, which all needed counter signing. I'm going to make friends with a rather large bottle of vodka tonight, that is all I am going to say about the matter!'

'Want a cup of tea?'

'I thought you would never ask!' Paul smiles.

As Paul and I sat in the office, we first saw Daniel's foot slowly shuffling into the office doorway, then a hand, and an arm, and first Daniel's elongated nose, and finally his full body was right in the doorway. Daniel would often walk slowly and carefully into other residents' bedrooms, and peer into the rooms like he had found some magical fantasy world behind each door. The look of fascination on his face would be intense, and he would often stay in the residents' rooms for hours on end, playing with numerous bed covers and small stuffed animals from time to time. Whatever took his fancy.

Paul shouted out to Daniel.

'Hello Dan mate.'

Daniel initially looked ahead. You could tell he heard Paul's shout but hadn't quite worked out where it had come from. He turns very slowly towards the nursing office to face us both.

'Oh..hello.'

'You all right Dan?'

'Yep.'

Dan starts to walk into the nursing office. Something on top of the medication fridge has taken his fancy, and he is focusing on it as he gently ushers himself into the office. There is a random selection of paper on top of the fridge; repositioning charts and diet and fluid charts. Daniel starts to pick these up and randomly move them from one side of the fridge to another, seemingly fascinated with their texture and appearance.

Paul and I let Daniel rearrange the office for a while. Daniel starts to pick up some of the nursing notes, Paul interjects quickly.

'Thank you Daniel, I need those, unless you're going to help me with them?'

Daniel looks confusedly at Paul.

'Well I uhh, hmmmmm yes.'

Daniel has one of the nursing files clutched in his hand, and a small vase in his other hand. Paul gently tries to take the nursing file off Daniel.

'Hey, fuck off will you, I need it!'

'Hey Daniel, I need to write my notes in this, can I just have this for one second please?'

'Nooooo, fuck off! I need it I tell you!'

Daniel grimaces, his eyes bulge, and he stares back out at Paul.

'Hey, Daniel.'

'What?'

'Can I have the file please? Here you are, why don't you take a look outside at the posters on the wall?'

Paul points towards some of the posters on the wall. Daniel lets out a semi sigh.

'Oh all right then.'

Daniel walks out of the nursing station, still clutching a small vase in his hand. He is stooped over, and walking incredibly slowly, one tiny half step at a time.

2-3 p.m.

Paul looks tired. He offers me a chair, and I sit down by him. His eyes say it all; he lets out a large sigh.

'What's up?' I ask meekly.

'Ah nothing mate, it's just I had a bit of bad news about a colleague of mine today. She was a great nurse...She's been sacked.'

'You got to watch yourself here, the carers have all the power.'

I didn't like to pry or push for any further information, but Paul was ready to tell me.

'Well mate, it all started like this; she was a night nurse, on this unit....'

Night shifts. There are important lessons to be learnt when doing night shifts. Apart from completely reversing your circadian rhythm and feeling like a zombie each morning and being more and being more detached from the world as you do more shifts, there are specific rules;

1. You do NOT sleep on night shifts.

2. You do **NOT** sleep on night shifts.

3. You do **NOT** sleep on night shifts.

And rule 4, if you were really wondering:

4. You do **NOT** sleep on night shifts.

Angela was in her mid sixties, close to retirement age, and had transferred from another nursing home recently as they no longer wished to employ her due to her being near a 'pensionable age'. She had many years of experience and had at one point run a small nursing home herself. She was perfectly able to handle herself and had the knowledge to back it up. She was short in stature, and had a small silvery-grey bob of hair, with deep brown eyes and a nice smile. She enjoyed a drink and would often socialise with the other nurses on the unit, and frequently drank them all under the table. She had travelled the world many times over, and had a real sense of what life was all about, and knew how to live it.

Angela had been working on the unit for five to six months and had had a previous run in with a younger carer who had accused her of being too 'bossy' and 'short' with the residents. Rather than approach Angela in a kind and considered way and ask her about her approaches the carer had decided to put in a formal complaint to the acting manager.

The carer was bad mouthing Angela in the smoking shelter and saying how she didn't like how she was treating the residents, being a little too 'rough' with them.

Paul never believed it for a second; Angela had over thirty years of experience in mental health, and she knew what she was doing. Any comments about being 'short' or 'bossy' would translate as 'assertive' and 'knowledgeable'. The carer was making big waves in the smoking shelter community, and this information had gradually seeped its way back to Angela through another nurse who had found out the allegations against her. Once Angela found out about what the carer was saying about her, she hit the roof. She often worked with this carer on nights and not once had the carer mentioned anything about it to her or said if she was unhappy. This seemed to be common practice in this home; the chain of command was irrelevant. If the carers had a problem with someone, they usually went straight to the top, and bypassed everyone else up the ladder.

Angela was no fool and the next time she was on shift with this carer she questioned her about it. The carer backed down almost immediately and began crying, denying the whole thing had even happened, telephoning her boyfriend to say how upset she was about the matter.

When Paul was on shift the next morning, Jennifer came up and accosted him and started to ask him questions about a particular night shift, and where the handover sheet was. The handover sheet was not found, and the acting manager went on to start asking about a particular resident and his usual behaviour on nights. His frequent behaviour would be to shuffle along on his bottom up and down the corridor, and sometimes he would wander. Paul had wondered what was going on, and he was immediately ordered to update all of the residents' risk assessments. When he asked if there was a problem, Jennifer simply stated 'there could be' in her vaguest tone.

Management would never bother the nurses unless there was a serious problem. This would often annoy some of the nurses as they frequently felt undervalued and had a low morale. Appraisals were never high on the list of priorities.

As Paul went down later that afternoon to get a print out from outside Jennifer's office, he spotted Angela sat outside, looking a little anxious.

'Angela! What are you doing here love?'

'Well would you believe it Paul, someone's dobbed me in for sleeping on nights!'

Paul looked flabbergasted.

'What! You're joking aren't you?! What the hell is this place coming to? Who was it, do you know?'

'Nope, no idea mate. It's ridiculous, it is, I've got to see Jennifer and be quizzed about it.' Angela looked heartbroken.

'Sorry to hear that Ange, listen if you need anything let me know, and I'll give you a ring later, see what the score is okay?'

'Yeah do that Paul, cheers mate.' Angela continued to look downbeat.

Paul described the scene of Angela being made to sit outside the manager's office like a naughty school kid.

According to the gossip and rumour mill of the smoking shelter Angela had been on a night shift, sat in the lounge area. A nurse (who normally works days) had come walking through the lounge area to get something and spotted Angela asleep in the lounge with her feet up on another chair. As the nurse had carried on through to the nursing office she spotted a resident on the floor shuffling along on his bottom. The nurse didn't say anything at the time, but quickly reported Angela to the management the following day.

Once this initial complaint had been filed, the management were then on a witch hunt, beginning to ask other carers who had worked with Angela, and demanding statements from them. One carer described the presence and force of management as very intimidating, making her do a statement or her 'job was on the line'. The carer made a statement, and told all the staff that it was a horrendous ordeal and she had felt like crying. They had sat her down in a small, cramped hot office and began asking her questions about Angela, and Jennifer had stated that she didn't believe what she was saying as she was looking 'quite flushed' and demanded her to think carefully about her answers.

It would later come out that her statement indicated that Angela was frequently 'bossy' and 'intimidating' to work for, despite telling the rest of the staff that she felt pressurised into making the statement.

Another carer had described that Angela was asleep and she felt 'frightened' and 'intimidated' to go wake her. If she was worried that Angela would not wake, then she should have surely been pro active in waking her. One carer had burst into tears even talking about it. She had stated that 'Angela will probably never speak to me again'. But they all agreed that they had to protect their own jobs.

Angela was being accused of sleeping for 'six hours at a time' whilst on a 12 hour night shift. Paul had never found any problems with Angela's work when he came in on the morning shift. If someone had been sleeping that long then there would not be any care needs met for the residents; one carer cannot successfully meet the needs on their own, despite the carer claiming that this is what she had to do, as Angela was either 'unwakeable' or too 'intimidating', depending on whose statement you read.

In the end they had five statements from various carers all saying that they had seen Angela sleep on at least one occasion, some describing the minute details of Angela placing her shoes and socks down on the floor beside her feet.

Paul had a feeling that Angela was given the sack because of her knowledge of the industry. This could be seen as a threat to the company as she would often assert her opinions on how things needed to be changed for the better to fall in line with care standards. The unit manager had already had a few dealings with Angela, and a rift had started to develop quite early on.

Angela had a week's leave, and by the time she came back, she was in the office, being read all the statements against her. They had even got a statement off the girl who had previously been talking about her in the smoking shelter who had cried when Angela had confronted her about the allegations made against her for being 'rough' and 'short' with some of the residents. Angela didn't have a chance. She was told she could appeal the decision, but otherwise she was out, and down the road. Angela decided for a few days on what to do. She was tired and didn't feel she had the energy to appeal and really take the company down a peg or two with some of the standards she felt were slipping. She took their decision without a fight, and left the company.

'And that's how it was' Paul said dejectedly. 'So just be careful mate, be very careful, they won't think anything of it to dob you in, for anything.'

I thought long and hard about what Paul had said. It made me think about working time directives. During the day each staff member was entitled to three breaks throughout the day: one morning twenty minute break (usually between 11 a.m. – 11.40 a.m.), one thirty minute break for lunch (usually between 1.30 p.m. – 2 p.m.), and one twenty minute break in the afternoon (usually between 3.30 p.m. – 4.40 p.m.). Night staff didn't have set break times but were often expected to work through a complete twelve hour shift with no break. I remember reading a few years ago that the Nursing Times was trying to look into this anomaly as it did not seem particularly fair, but I haven't heard anything regarding this.

The phone rings, a shrill ring. Paul was really starting to show the the stresses of the day on his wrinkled brow. He picks the phone up. A few moments later he puts the phone back down and turns to me.

'You won't believe this...we have an admission coming in this afternoon! It was Sally, she said they have an emergency assessment from another care home where this chap is, and they want him moved to us straight away. He is at high risk of absconding, and where he is they don't seem to be able to deal with him very well at all, seems like they're going to ship him onto us.'

'Oh right okay, what do we need to do then?'

'The room's ready, we just need to settle him in and start up all the paperwork. He has four daughters and two of them are a nightmare according to Sally, bordering on the psychotic, so that will be a lot of fun.'

'What's his name?'

'Ian...Ian Korvlov.'

Ian Korvlov, sixty five, used to be in the plastering business. Later in his life he ran his own self employed plastering business, having four daughters who doted on their father. Ian's wife died a few years ago on this unit, and since then Ian's deterioration had been increasing. Diagnosed with vascular dementia, his short term memory was getting worse, often forgetting things a few moments later. He walked, but was unsteady, and required a walking stick at all times. The daughters started to find their dad frequently on the floor in his home or in the garden, and he would often leave his keys on the inside of the front door, so the daughters couldn't get hold of him to check if he was okay. Ian had worked hard his entire life, hard enough to allow him to retire at fifty and enjoy the trappings of a very successful career, with a string of exotic holidays and sports cars, including Ferraris and Porsches.

There were a few occasions when Ian was found in the middle of his local high street without him realising where he was or how he could get home. Ian was originally from the midlands, and spoke with a semi thick Wolverhampton accent. He could self care to a degree, but would often get confused with the stages of getting dressed and would sometimes forget to put on clothes, or wear his pyjamas over the top of his normal daily clothing.

The family despised one another. Two of the daughters had power of attorney for their dad, which caused a massive rift between the other two daughters. Ian still had a girlfriend, who wasn't really liked by the daughters but they appreciated that the girlfriend made their dad happy, so had to put up with her. The daughters were seen to be fighting and bickering over their dying mother over money countless times whilst she was on this unit.

Paul begins to get a file ready in preparation with various bits of documentation.

Paul didn't have much time to sort out his documentation as only moments later the phone rang again. It was reception.

'Here we go then,' Paul whispered under his breath.

I followed Paul slowly up the corridor. Bob was walking up the corridor, still salivating profusely. Paul took a small tissue out of Bob's shirt pocket and quickly wiped the saliva away. Bob tried to look up at Paul as best he could, and mumbled under his breath. He began to walk away from Paul and back down the corridor. This would be Bob's usual activity for most of the afternoon. At times Bob could grab hold of you incredibly tightly and not let go for some time, grimacing and shouting at you, but his strength was starting to go, so you could wait it out and Bob would resume to his normal wandering self. But for anyone who didn't know about Bob, it could be quite scary.

I remember on my first placement area, I went to get an elderly gentleman a tissue. As soon as I gestured to give him the tissue, both hands immediately locked onto my wrist, and he wouldn't let go. There was no one about to shout to, and I panicked. Sweat was pouring from me as I tried desperately to free myself from the vice like grip. Eventually I managed it, but from that day onwards I was always wary. You assume just because people are elderly they don't have much strength. That myth is completely wrong, and it was proven to me that day, and became a lesson to me that I have taken with me to every placement area and workplace.

As I was following Paul up the corridor, I could already see two large stocky men at the door of the unit, dressed in what looked like army combats and t-shirts. These were the ambulance drivers.

Paul opened the door, and one of the men walked in. The other, who was stood back a little, gestured to the man behind him.

'Come on Ian, right through here.'

Ian slowly walked through the unit door, looking a little confused. Ian was wearing a dark blue jacket, clutching at his gnarled walking stick. He wore square gold rimmed glasses which had an inch of dust on them, and his white hair was straight as a razor, curled off to the left at the front. He had kind eyes, and a nice smile.

'What, through here? Is this the way out?' Ian spoke with a very heavy Wolverhampton accent.

'Yes, this is the way out,' the ambulance driver said half heartedly.

'Right you are,' Ian replied.

Ian took one look at Paul and I, and for a moment paused, then asked inquisitively;

'Is this the way out fellas?'

'Yes!' Paul and I reply in unison.

'Ahh, okay lads, just asking, see me right will you?'

We walk down with Ian. One of the ambulance drivers hands Paul a large clear plastic bag which is full with medication.

'This is all he came with, and all the paperwork we have with him is in there, okay?'

'Righto,' Paul says.

The ambulance drivers quickly leave the unit, slamming the door shut behind them.

We continued to walk down the corridor with Ian.

'Would you like a cup of tea Ian?' Paul asked.

'Oh I wouldn't say no to a coffee actually.'

'Okay, no problem, do you take sugar?'

'Yes, just one please, and don't make it too hot.'

'Okay. Jack are you okay to show Ian to his room? Right down the bottom of the corridor, last door on the left.'

'Sure.'

I continue to walk Ian down the corridor as Paul goes off to make Ian a drink. Ian is looking at all the pictures on the wall and taking everything in in his new environment. Bob walks past us slowly. Ian stops, and looks a little confused.

'Hey there, what's this fella's name then?'

'Bob.'

'Bob?'

'Bob,' I say.

'Oh right, well he looks like he could do with a hand, is he all right?'

'Oh he's fine,' I reply.

Ian outstretches a hand to shake Bob's. I immediately intervene.

'Oh it's okay Ian, he's fine, he just likes to walk up and down the corridor, I wouldn't shake his hand if I was you.'

'Well I was just trying to be friendly, but okay, if that's the way you want to play it, then I won't.'

'Okay, let's just see your room first okay?'

'Show me the way then!'

We carry on down to the bottom of the corridor, and I show Ian his room. The room is nice and airy, and well carpeted. Ian sits down in the chair by the bed, and looks a little perplexed at his new surroundings.

'Well this is a nice building all right, isn't it?' Ian exclaims excitedly.

'Sure is.'

'How many rooms are in here then?'

'Eighty in total, but twenty on this unit.'

'Twenty! Wow, this must have cost quite a bit of money to do up then!'

'Yeah, I would have thought so.'

I can hear Paul singing down the corridor as he makes his way to Ian's room. He walks into the room and presents Ian with a large blue plastic mug of coffee.

'Here you go Ian, nice cup of coffee for you!'

'Well that's smashing fellas, thank you for that, you do look after me you two don't you!'

'We try our best!' Paul says.

Ian takes a small sip of his coffee, and smiles.

'Smashing.'

Paul leans over to Ian.

'Listen Ian, you have got your own toilet just in that room over there, and this is your bedroom. You have a TV and your own wardrobe, all nice and to yourself.'

'Smashing, yep.'

It wasn't clear if Ian was taking this information in. Paul was doing his best to explain it all to him.

'Shall we leave you for a minute then Ian, and pop back a bit later?'

Ian looks up at both of us.

'Yep, okay fellas, let me have this coffee then I'll join you.'

'Okay, Ian, we will see you in a bit then?'

'Yep.'

Paul and I leave Ian with his cup of coffee, and walk back up the corridor to the nursing office.

'Let's just see how long the pleasantries last eh?' Paul says to me.

Paul starts sorting out the medication for Ian, and the paperwork, going through some of the notes. The notes state that Ian can become quite agitated and aggressive and has been known to hit out at some residents, and could be sexually inappropriate to some of the female carers. The advice is that two carers dealt with Ian at all times, particularly when trying to encourage him to get dressed and washed in the morning.

Ian has vascular dementia and his short term memory loss could be quite severe. Ian had been a huge smoker in his day. The experts were linking a lot more cases of vascular dementia with heavy smoking, as smoking constricts the blood vessels, and vascular dementia means the brain isn't getting enough blood supply to it.

Paul begins filling in some of the documentation. One of the most important jobs of the day would be to fax across a registration form to the local GP, so that they could register the resident on their system. Other than that, basic observations had to be taken: pulse, blood pressure, and temperature, and an entry in the notes stating how the resident was presenting upon admission. Other than that, just as Paul had started to do, a bit of TLC and a good cup of tea or coffee.

It would often take a few days for a resident to acclimatise to a new environment and surroundings, often a very difficult step for someone to take, someone who is already confused and unfamiliar with their surroundings. Add to the mix that they are now in an environment where there are so many different residents with different stages of dementia, it was always a bit of a juggling act as to whether residents would get on with one another, but this would also be a skill when assessing someone to see if they were suitable for the unit.

I began to hear some heavy feet walking up the corridor, shuffling a little, and then a big loud 'thunk'. I walk outside to where the noise was emanating from. It was Ian. Ian was no longer wearing his jacket, or his shirt. He was walking up the corridor, with his walking stick in his hand.

'Ian! Are you alright?'

'No, not really, I'm trying to find the way out.'

'They're going to be making some afternoon drinks soon, and you haven't got your shirt on!'

'I've got plenty of shirts, I just want to get out, just show me the way will you?'

'I can't show you the way, they're going to get drinks in a moment.'

'Just run me up the road will you? It will only take you five minutes, I'll see you right I promise.'

'Ian, I can't, I have to stay here till eight o'clock.'

'Eight! Your having a laugh aren't you?'

'No seriously, I have to stay here, don't you want to put a shirt on?'

'No, not right now.'

I could hear a noise behind me, some more shuffling of feet. It was Mindy, trying to get past and go to the toilet again.

'Norman! Norman!'

'Please help me Norman!'

I turn to the direction of Mindy. She is by the large windows again, holding her hand outstretched. I grab it, and take her across the corridor past the windows. She stops dead in her tracks, and stares at Ian.

'Who's he?'

'Ian' I mouth clearly to Mindy.

'Ian.'

'Yes, Ian.'

'Take him away will you, he's got no shirt on!'

Mindy was not very keen on some of the male residents, and usually had run ins with Bob up and down the corridor on a daily basis.

'Go on, get away will you?' she shouted directly at Ian.

Ian stared at Mindy, almost fascinated by her, and smiled.

'I'm not doing any harm love, can you get past me?'

'Go on get away will you, or I'll hit you!'

'Hang on love, there's no need for that, I'm just trying to get home that's all.'

Mindy was getting more and more agitated. I was stood right in the middle of them, fearing that things were going to get a little more heated.

'Come on, get away will you, you look like a paddy, fuck off you paddy.'

Ian smiled.

'I'm a what?'

'Paddy, a fucking paddy, now get away before I hit you, you bastard.'

Ian continued to try and appease the situation.

'Listen love, there's no need for that, I am not a paddy. I like the look of you, but don't call me names, there is no need for that.'

'Go on, shoo will you.'

'Listen you, I will give you what for in a minute, talking like that.'

Ian starts to raise his fists and grimaces.

I try to steer Mindy around Ian, before the situation turns to fisticuffs. Ian is just staring at Mindy with amazement. Mindy is coaxed around Ian and I show her where the toilet is.

'Right thank you, now make sure you get rid of him before I come back OK!'

Mindy slams the toilet door shut, and I walk back to Ian.

'Don't worry about her Ian, she gets a little grumpy.'

'Oh, okay, well I was just trying to be friendly with her, but she doesn't seem to like that, seems quite a nasty little woman.'

'Ian, shall we just come and sit in the quiet lounge for a bit?'

I walk Ian into the quiet lounge and sit him down. He sits looking at me with a blank expression on his face.

'Ian, what's the matter then, what can I help with?'

'Well, I want to get out, I need to get home, my daughters are going to be there, and I haven't got time to stay here.'

'Okay, do you know where you are Ian?'

Ian smiles at me.

'Well I've got a very good idea.'

'Okay, where do you think you are?'

'Well, I don't know, but it's a nice place.'

'Ian, you're in a nursing home.'

There was a moments silence. Ian looks to be thinking these words over in his head.

'Get out!!' he smiles.

'Honestly.'

'Honestly? You're having a laugh aren't you?'

'You were bought here because your daughters were concerned that you were having a lot of falls at home and that you were posing a considerable risk to yourself.'

'Falls? I wasn't having any falls, that's rubbish that is, complete rubbish, I need to get home.'

I was trying my best to give an open and honest approach to Ian. Grounding someone to their reality of time and place wasn't always easy.

'I've got a garden to attend to you know, I haven't got time to spend it here with you, as much as I like you.'

'Ian, this is your home now, we are going to look after you, and there is a garden here that you might like to have a look at tomorrow.'

'I've got my own garden thank you very much, I don't need another one.'

'Ian, I don't quite think you understand where you are.'

'I do, you've told me, but I'm not interested I'm afraid. Can you run me up the road? It will only take you a few minutes'

'I can't Ian, I have to stay here until eight o'clock.'

'Oh, well what time is it now?'

'It's about half past two.'

'Oh, that's quite a long time to wait, I don't think I can wait that long.'

'Ian, why don't you stay here and have some tea with us later?'

'I can get my own tea at home, it will be waiting for me, I can't wait here for it you know!'

I was running out of ideas. Everything I had been taught at university I was struggling to try and remember. This was one of the hardest parts of the job, when residents clearly had enough awareness about them to want to leave the premises, and not be interested in anything you had to say. I remember one of my fellow colleagues had tried distracting their patients by trying to incorporate bizarre statements from movies to try and help ease the situation. He sometimes worked a few miracles and managed to calm his residents down a little. I decided to go for it. I could only really think of a few to start with. The first one was Wall Street.

Ian continued to stare at me.

'What are you doing now then? Are you going to take me up the road?'

I tried a quote.

'I can't I'm afraid, I'm *just kicking ass and taking names* Ian.'

'You're what ? Well why are you doing that? I'm not interested in any of that, you can do what you like!'

I decided to try the film Taken, starring Liam Neeson.

'Ian.'

'Yes.'

'*I have a particular set of skills you know.*'

'Do ya? What like?'

I was confused, so I blurted out:

'Things like espionage and weaponry.'

Ian took just a few seconds to process this information and without flinching spoke again.

'Well we don't need those at the minute, I just need you to run me up the road.'

This new tactic wasn't working; I wasn't getting anywhere with Ian at all. I had tried reality orientation, I had tried distraction. Paul suddenly came to my rescue. He appeared at the door with a medicine pot in his hand and a spoon. He had been listening to our conversation.

'Ian!'

Ian turns round and looks at Paul.

'What?'

'I've just got your tablets for you.'

'Have you? Oh okay then.'

Paul gradually popped a half milligram of Lorazepam onto the spoon and held it close to Ian's mouth, Ian immediately took the spoon off Paul and took the tablet.

Paul gave him a small glass of water, and Ian swallowed the tablet almost immediately.

'Thanks.'

I remember a charge nurse telling me that sometimes you simply had to go for the medication route straight away. I used to have long conversations with nurses about how we should be more patient centred, spending time and talking with these people, but they all argued that it was fine in a lecture theatre, but on the ward, sometimes you had to medicate immediately, and worry about the rest later. Medication had its place, and it wasn't always to be in last position.

I had taken this to heart a little as I was quite opposed to giving people medication just for the sake of it, but I was now beginning to realise that it did have a place, and I wasn't always cut out to be talking my way out of situations, as sometimes no matter what you said, it wouldn't make a difference; if a resident was agitated and restless, you could say anything and it wouldn't change a thing, however I was still a firm believer that medication should always be the last resort, and we should at least try everything we have got before we go down that route. In the hospitals they appeared very quick to dismiss any kind of talking therapy.

'How much will it take then?'

'How much will what take?'

'To run me up the road. I don't like seeing people out of pocket, and you have been good to me, so I want to see you right.'

'Honestly Ian, I can't take your money off you, I need to stay here and work.'

'No one will have to know! I won't tell anyone, but I want to see you right okay?'

'Ian.'

'Yes?'

'You used to be a plasterer didn't you?'

'I did yes, what's that got to do with it?'

'Well I was just wondering about it that's all, hey would you like another drink?'

'I've just had one, but go on then, and then I'll have to get going.'

'Okay, coffee and one sugar wasn't it?'

'Yep, that's the one.'

'Okay.'

I quickly leap out of my seat and go to the kitchen area. I was glad to get out of the room, it was becoming quite intense, and I wasn't getting anywhere at all. It was quite a challenge. I remembered how easy the lecturers had made it look with their examples of the difficult patient. It was certainly not so easy when you were in the hot seat. It was quite logical that Ian would want to leave, he probably didn't have any idea where he was, and now all these strangers just kept wanting to make him cups of coffee.

I walked back into the quiet lounge and placed Ian's drink on the table in front of him.

Ian looked at me attentively.

'Right then, what are we going to do?'

'Well later we are going to have something to eat, do you fancy sticking around for that?'

'Not really.'

'It's free you know!'

'I don't care really, I want to get back home and see to my family.'

'Your daughter will probably visit sometime this evening.'

'She won't; I've got to see her back at home.'

Ian suddenly started to get a little angry.

'Listen, I've known you a number of years, and this is the way you treat me? I have been very good to you in the past, and all I ask of you is just this one favour, just to run me up the road. Me and you are going to fall out over this, and I don't want to fall out, I just want you to help me out, like I did all those years ago.'

'Ian, I know, but I simply cannot do it today, I think you should stay here today, and we can look at going out tomorrow okay?'

'Tomorrow?'

'Yes tomorrow, I promise.'

'Are you sure? Because I trust you, and if we shake on it, then that's a bond, and you will have to make good on your word.'

'I will, I promise.'

Ian outstretches a hand to me and shakes it.

'Okay then, tomorrow, but I will be checking on you and coming to see you.'

Ian smiles.

'Yes, no problem, now are you going to get a shirt on ready for tea a bit later?'

'A shirt?'

'Yes'

'Well, I could do I suppose, now then, where's the toilet round here?'

'Straight out this door and round to the left, first door on the left.'

'Come and show me will you?'

Ian slowly stands up and walks with his walking stick around the corner. I show him the toilet door with its clear signs on it and bid him good day.

'Will you be okay now Ian?'

'Yes I'll be fine now, where's the light switch?'

I switch the light on for him.

'Marvellous, yep, I'll be fine now okay.'

'Okay Ian, I'll just be outside.'

'Okay.'

I shut the door behind Ian, and wait patiently outside. Ian was seeming to respond well to the odd bit of distraction, but if he was going to continually ask to leave the premises then we would have to do something. Ian was not under section under the Mental

Health Act, which would normally allow you to legally detain people. However if someone was continually asking to leave, then there were other legal frameworks that could be put in place to provide these holding powers. The deprivation of liberty safeguards (DOLS) could be initiated in order to see that people like Ian were kept here on this unit. We were keeping him here for his best interests as he posed a considerable risk to himself or others if he was to continue living at his own home. This would require a separate assessment that the nursing team would have to fill in here, and then an independent assessor would come in to assess if they thought Ian was being detained for the right reasons. You had to be very careful in healthcare that everything was being done for the resident's best interests, and had documentation to back everything up.

I can hear Ian flushing the toilet, and moments later he comes out. I start walking him down to his room, and once there, find his shirt for him which is draped over the back of the chair.

He puts his shirt back on with my help, and I do the buttons up for him.

'There, that's better isn't it?'

'Yep.'

'Now then, what would you like to do now? Would you like to sit here in your room and watch a bit of telly, or join the others in the lounge?'

'I'll just sit here, I'm fine actually.'

'Okay.'

I put the TV on for Ian. He seems a lot more relaxed now, and he smiles at me.

'I must say this is a lovely place here isn't it, how many rooms are here?'

'Twenty rooms on this unit, but eighty in the whole building.'

'Wow that is a lot isn't it, I'm very impressed with the place indeed.'

'Yeah, sure is.'

'Now then, I need to go to the toilet.'

'You have just been Ian!'

'I haven't! Just point me in the right direction and I'll find it.'

'There's a toilet right here Ian, you have your own en suite bathroom, it says toilet on it.'

'Ah, well that's good isn't it, is that extra then for that?'

'No, totally free of charge Ian, don't worry about it.'

'Oh, I'll use that in a minute then, thanks.'

'No problem at all. Is that everything now then ? You're all settled?'

'Yep, that will be fine thanks.'

'I'll be back later then.'

'Back later.' The mantra for all nurses that should be engraved on our gravestone's. How many times would we be back 'later'? It just seemed to roll off the tongue, but there would always be things to do, and tasks to be involved with. It was already going to be quite a struggle to spend time with the residents, and grab precious time with them. But I was going to do my best to make as much time as possible, no matter how difficult things got.

Ian took one last look at me, and smiles.

'You're a nice fella you are, you can come back again any time.'

3–4 p.m.

Sharon is organising large pots of tea and coffee, arranging all the beakers and mugs ready onto the trolley. She is busily wheeling it into the lounge area where I was stood for the afternoon drinks.

'Right baby, let me sort these drinks out for you and you can help out.'

About half of the residents could drink by themselves, the others required assistance. Some of the residents would require their drinks to be thickened as they were at further risk of choking. The industry standard Thick n' Easy was used to help with this, and I was familiar with this from my student days. Large blue tubs, with a blue plastic spoon inside. It was essentially starch, and a few scoops of this added to any drink did what it said on the tin, it thickened it. It could thicken to a consistency allowing you to stand a spoon upright.

Sharon was well versed in this routine. She was making up drinks, adding sugar, stirring, and placing the drinks in front of the residents who could drink for themselves.

Sharon passed me a small beaker with a lid on. The beakers were a pale beige colour and you could position a small clear lid on if required, just like a beaker a baby would have. This allowed more accurate flow of liquid for the residents to consume.

'Right, this is Edward's coffee, he probably won't want any, but just go and see if you can get a few sips down him. I think Emma has gone in there just to try and see if she can encourage him to eat anything, we're just keeping an eye on him every hour really, okay?'

'Yeah, sure.'

I walked up past Edward's room. Emma was in there feeding him. She shouted out to me.

'Jack, Edward's not sounding so good you know.'

'What's the matter?' I say.

'He is sounding very chesty.'

I walk in to see Edward. He is sat up in bed, and turns towards me.

'How are you Edward? Are you all right?'

'Half left,' he replies.

He was sounding very wheezy and crackly as he breathed. A bubbling sound was erupting each and every time he was breathing.

Emma turns to Edward.

'Edward, are you in any pain?'

'Noooo.'

There was a long pause.

'I feel funny though.'

'I'll go get Paul' I volunteer.

I quickly walk out of the door, and see Paul in the opposite room with another resident. I beckon him over, and he comes walking up to me.

'I think you need to see Edward again, his chest is quite crackly.'

Paul comes racing over and walks into Edward's room and we both stand over him, and listen once more to the crackles.

'Has he eaten much today Emma?' Paul asks.

'Hardly anything. He is only taking small sips of his drink, he refused his lunch which is unusual for him, and seems to have been slipping in and out of consciousness at times' Emma states.

'The doctor put him on Ciprofloxacin this morning for a urine infection, and that is a strong antibiotic to cover a chest infection too. She did say he sounded a little wheezy this morning. If he's not eating or drinking, and not very responsive, we may have to put him on the LCP. Let's keep an eye on him anyway.'

The LCP is the Liverpool Care Pathway, a document used in the end stages of life, and is a framework which professionals can utilise in the care of the dying patient. It is an ongoing document and people can often be put on the pathway, and also taken off if they improve. It is not always as clear cut as the documentation suggests. It provides guidance in pain management, and in terms of nursing notes, the pathway takes over as the main focus of all documentation. It is good practice to put someone on this pathway if you thought they were at the end stages. Not everyone went on the pathway, as some deaths could be sudden.

'I'll go ring the family,' Paul said to me.

It was also good practice to alert family members to any considerable change in a resident's presentation. Paul walked back into the nursing office and began thumbing through Edwards notes to get the contact details of his nearest relative, his wife.

I am standing over Edward, listening to his increasingly loud breaths and crackling sounds. I check his catheter bag. It is draining, but still very dark red and small bits are floating in it. Many patients who are dying have 'noisy respirations'. The sounds often come from retained secretions in the pharynx and the upper respiratory tree.

'Edward, can you hear me?'

Edward is lying on his side, but he is now not responding to me or Emma any more. Suddenly Jennifer comes walking through to us.

'Hi, so what's the trouble then?'

She checked him over, listened to his breathing, and turned to me.

'Is he on the LCP?'

'Not yet' I state. 'Paul is just ringing the wife now.'

'I would put him on it anyway, if he's not responsive or eating much it won't hurt, we can always take him off it if he improves.'

The main areas to look for when considering to put someone on the pathway is loss of consciousness, or a considerable lack or decline in diet and fluid intake over a number of days.

Paul comes rushing back into Edward's room.

He and Jennifer have a brief chat, and Paul explains the wife is on the way with the daughter.

Paul turns to me and whispers 'I don't think he's got long left you know, his legs are starting to mottle already.'

Hands and feet may often become blotchy and purplish. This mottling may slowly work its way up the arms and legs. It was quite common to become unresponsive and for people to have their eyes open or semi-open but not see their surroundings.

Edward was going to die. I started to feel very hot and slightly dizzy. I was just speaking to Edward not moments ago and now I was being told that he could be in the end stages. I had never witnessed a death before.

A few moments later there is a loud bang from the entrance door to the corridor. An older lady with bright white hair and a younger lady with black hair come walking down the corridor. They approach me and Paul who are standing in the corridor. Paul looks quite solemn, and ushers them into the room, explaining how he has been.

'Take as much time as you like, and just give us a shout if you need anything.'

The wife and daughter nod in unison, walk into Edward's room, and shut the door. I follow Paul down to the nursing office. He starts writing an entry in the LCP about how Edward is. It is good practice to write regular entries, and you are prompted to make an entry every twelve and every four hours, marking any changes in the resident's presentation, but you could also write an entry whenever you felt it necessary. The pathway took over from the patient's main notes and became the only documentation you needed.

'Do you want a coffee Paul?'

'I'd love a tea, milk no sugar.'

I walk out of the nursing station and down the corridor towards the kitchen. Just as I get to the kitchen door, the alarm goes off again, and I can hear the faint click of a room door being opened. Edward's daughter is rushing out and running down the corridor.

She comes running up to me. Paul has also leapt out of the nursing office.

'I think he's in pain.'

Paul and I walk back up to Edward's room. He is still breathing very heavily, and very crackly, but now appears to be flinching a little and there is a slight whimpering in his voice every few moments. Paul slowly places a hand gently on Edward's stomach, and he flinches and shouts out.

'He is on a Matrifen patch for pain, but I think he might need to go on a syringe driver at this stage.'

His daughter looks at Paul, confused.

'Just to help with the pain relief a little more, we can give him some morphine which will take the edge off a little.'

His daughter nods. She has a small tear forming in her left eye. Paul and I walk out of the room and Paul turns to me.

'We need to go get Jennifer, this guy needs a syringe driver in place asap.'

A syringe driver is a small portable device which is battery driven. An infusion pump is used to give medication subcutaneously via a syringe, usually over a twenty four hour period. I had heard about them before, but never witnessed one in action.

Paul puts the phone down in the nursing office.

'Jennifer is on her way, she will help show you the syringe driver. I'm not sure about it myself, it's been a while, and to be honest I haven't done the new training for it'

'Okay,' I say nervously.

I sit with Paul in the nursing office. I can hear the carers talking in the lounge area with some of the residents. Another loud banging door, and I hear Jennifer's voice from afar, saying something to the carers and a resident. She arrives at the nursing office, and turns to me.

'Okay, what's been happening then?'

Paul turns to Jennifer.

'We just had the daughter in, and I have been to see Edward. He is looking a lot more pained in his expression, his stomach hurts to the touch, and he is sounding a lot more crackly. He is getting a little agitated at times.'

'Syringe driver it is then.'

Jennifer turns to me.

'You can do this one.'

I gulp, and am very aware of a few beads of sweat appearing on my forehead.

'If you can show me.'

'No problem, it will be a good learning curve for you.'

Paul steps up.

'Right, I will leave you to it then, if that's alright?'

'Yeah, we will be fine,' Jennifer says.

Paul walks out of the nursing office, handing Jennifer the nursing keys, and Jennifer comes in and sits down next to me and puts a large plastic box down on the table.

'Right, we need Edward's end of life drugs.'

The end of life drugs were to help someone in their last days or hours to be pain free and comfortable. They would often be ordered in advance when the doctor thought that the patient was likely to be deteriorating and would need them soon. This of course was not always predictable, people rarely fit into neat little boxes, so this was not always the case, but best practice and experience often meant that these drugs were on hand at the right time.

Common end of life drugs

Midazolam - Anticonvulsant and a skeletal muscle relaxant, used to try and relax and make patients much calmer and less agitated during end stages.

Hyosciene butyl bromide - Antispasmodic, and primarily used in this instance to reduce secretions in the lung.

Diamorphine - Synthesized from morphine. An analgesic, used as a stronger pain relief.

Water for injections was also used to dilute the mix of these drugs. Not all these drugs needed to be used together, it would depend on how the patient was presenting.

Jennifer got Edward's end of life drugs and spread them out on the table. She got a large orange book labelled 'controlled drugs' and put this down in front of me.

'Right, we're going to give all three of these drugs, so best get writing.'

For each controlled drug it needs two qualified nurses to sign the documentation to say you were going to give it. This ensured everything was accurately checked and the right amounts were going to be administered. It would also make sure that there would be nothing untoward going on with the drugs in question.

The drugs you were dealing with were valuable property and had to be dealt with in a professional and safe manner. At any one time there could be thousands of pounds worth of medication in the nurse's possession on the unit.

I had to document the drug, the amount, and what time and date it was given, and then sign it, and then Jennifer had to counter sign.

'Right, get the ampoules out and start drawing them up,' Jennifer said.

I look over to the pile of drugs that are in a small plastic bag, and in lots of white boxes. I begin opening up the boxes, to find very small glass ampoules with each drug inside. The glass ampoules were smaller than your little finger. They reminded me of a tiny bowling alley skittle. They had a very small dot engraved onto the side where the glass was made a little weaker. This was the 'breaking point'. You had to push carefully away from you at this point on the ampoule in order to break it open, and then begin to draw up the liquid with the needle and syringe.

Often people would cut themselves on these small ampoules. I began to break some of the ampoules open. My syringe and needle were on the desk in front of me.

I attached my needle to the syringe, and unsheathed the needle. The needle was quite long. I then put the needle into the ampoule and began to draw back slowly on the syringe and suck up the medication out of the ampoule. You had to have very nimble fingers to be able to do this all in one fluid motion. Jennifer was watching me carefully.

'You need to tip the ampoules upside down and very carefully draw back,' she said.

It had been too long since I had done anything like this in my training; sometimes there are areas that you just were not exposed to. Mental health was so varied and wide ranging that you simply couldn't be involved in all skills and experiences in your three years training as a mental health nurse.

'Right up, they won't spill,' Jennifer urged me.

I tipped the ampoule upside down, and I had my needle still in the bottle. The ampoules were cleverly designed, and the liquid did not tip out, but I still had some trouble trying to get the liquid out. I carefully withdrew back on my syringe, allowing the needle to suck up the remaining liquid. My hands were trembling, and the needle was darting about inside the ampoule as

I nervously tried desperately to suck up the last remaining amounts.

'Don't worry, take your time, it took me a good half an hour to get it right when I first did this,' Jennifer gently assured me.

'It is really fiddly,' I say.

'Yeah, what you have to remember is just to take your time, and be careful, we don't want you stabbing yourself with a needle!'

'No, we sure don't!'

I carefully suck up all the remaining liquid, and carry onto the next ampoule, as Jennifer instructs me. We gradually work through all the medication and check it all off as we go along. An ampoule of water is then also mixed with the syringe full of medication. I could feel myself breaking into a sweat by the time I had got everything into the syringe.

The syringe had to have precisely 17ml of total fluid in it. You knew what your ampoules contained in mls, and whatever the difference, you had to add that amount with water, to make it up to 17ml and dilute the mixture. If you were using 3 ml of hyosciene, and 1ml of midazolam, you would require 13ml of water to add to this, to make the complete syringe, ready for the driver.

We then had to load the syringe onto the syringe driver. The syringe driver basically allowed the syringe to sit on top of a digital box and gradually, very slowly push the syringe gradually over a twenty four hour period, therefore slowly administering the mix of medication into the resident over this time frame. I clipped the syringe into place and it made a few whistles and beeps at me, and it was ready to go.

Jennifer then attached another smaller needle which had a very long tube with it onto the syringe. The small needle would be inserted into the resident and the medication would flow through the tube, the needle, and into the resident.

'Right, let's go see him then, we're all set.'

I walk up to Edward's room with Jennifer. I was thinking to myself, I really hope she is not expecting me to insert the needle into Edward, with his family being there. I was really starting to panic. I really felt like I didn't want to go through this procedure ever again. It had felt like such a complex and stressful procedure.

We walk into Edward's room. The wife and daughter are sat by Edward. Edward appears to be in the same state, he is very crackly, and his eyes are shut. He is still breathing but it appearing more laboured.

Jennifer slowly puts the syringe driver down by Edward's legs, and gently pinches a bit of skin from Edward's upper thigh.

'Slight scratch Edward.'

She inserts the needle quickly and efficiently into the area. A slight wince comes from Edward. She pushes the button on the syringe driver, and it whirs into action.

'What's that for ?' the daughter asks.

'It's just to manage his pain and any secretions or agitation, and delivers the medication very slowly over a 24 hour period,' Jennifer answers assuringly.

The daughter just nods, along with the wife. Jennifer and I walk out of Edward's room, and Jennifer turns to me.

'We won't need that syringe driver long at all, he is quite mottled now, it probably won't be more than a few hours.'

'I'm sorry I was so nervous, it's just so...fiddly'

'Don't worry about it, you'll be fine, it just takes a lot of getting used to, but it's important, and you can't afford to make any mistakes, just take as long as you need, you will be fine.'

And with that Jennifer walks off the unit once more.

Paul comes round the corner and into the nursing office.

'How did you get on then?'

'Well, it's quite a complicated procedure, but the syringe driver is in place now and the family have been updated. Jennifer doesn't think he has long though.'

'Right,' Paul says.

There is another bang of the door, on the far side of the unit. Paul and I both look at each other, and walk around the corner of the nursing office. There is a group of people coming down the corridor; at least six or seven.

Paul walks confidently up to the group to meet them half way, and I trail behind nervously.

The front member of the group is a younger girl with short black hair.

'Hi, we have come to see Edward.'

Paul ushers them towards Edward's room. They all go in one by one, solemnly. Paul is very calm and collected, and gradually shuts the door behind them. Edward had a very large family that included at least five sons and daughters, and grandchildren too. I had never seen so many people walk into one small room.

'Just let me know if you need anything.'

Paul walks back down the corridor towards me.

'Time for another cup of tea I think, today is going to be a long day.'

Paul walks off to the kitchen area, and I go and sit in the nursing office. I can still hear Sharon finishing off the drinks in the lounge.

I can hear some shuffling outside the nursing office. Bob was still wandering the corridors. His head was firmly fixed in a downwards trajectory. This could often be a side effect of large amounts of anti psychotic medication. Bob was on a lot of Risperidone, the only antipsychotic licensed for use with dementia, which could vastly increase the risk of a stroke with increased use.

Bob would often get very agitated and verbally aggressive, but usually he would simply walk the corridors in between meal times. His salivating was a common side effect of antipsychotic medication.

Bob started to walk into the office area around me. He looked down at me with his dark brown eyes.

'Yeah heheyeye mmmmmmmmm.'

He started moving some of the files around on the desk, gently trying to rearrange them.

'How you doing Bob?' I ask.

A very large saliva trail is emanating from Bob's mouth. It's getting longer and longer. I quickly reach for a small tissue and wipe the saliva away from his mouth. He starts moving a few more files around, and then sits down on the chair in the office. After a few seconds he stands up. He sits down again, then stands up.

I stare transfixed at this behaviour. He appears to be very restless, but this is his normal presentation. After watching him stand up and sit down a good half a dozen times, Bob eventually starts walking towards the corridor again and out of the nursing office. I can hear him whispering to himself, but I cannot make any of it out in a logical coherent manner.

'Hehehehehehe   msssmmsmsmssm   yes mmsmssmsmsm.'

Bob carries on walking up the corridor. Another saliva bead is starting to form around his lips as he exits the office area.

Paul comes bounding back with two fresh cups of coffee in his hand.

'Righto, time to do the notes then, do you want to give me a hand?'

'Yeah, sure.'

Paul grabs the notes for all twenty residents, and I follow in after him into the lounge area with the cups of tea.

Around this time of day was the best time to do the nursing notes. This was one of the main duties of the day for a qualified nurse. One entry in each of the residents' nursing notes had to be documented each day. A typical example of this could be anything like:

'Elsie up, washed and dressed this morning and assisted to lounge area after breakfast. Accepted good diet and fluid intake and has remained settled in mood in the lounge area watching television and interacting with the other residents. Daughter visited this evening.'

An entry had to be entered every night too. You could make as many additional entries as you wished. If something out of the ordinary happened or someone was getting particularly aggressive or there was an incident (such as a fall), then another entry would often be made. Many of the notes hadn't been updated for a number of months. A few didn't have current pictures of the residents' faces, some didn't even have any pictures at all. Pictures should be updated at least once a year, so that any new members of staff working on the unit could easily recognise each resident.

Paul walked into the lounge area to the far table, and stacked the residents notes high. He split them off into two separate piles, and I begin working my way through some of the notes.

Each of the notes should detail essential information such as the next of kin, funeral arrangements and funeral directors they wished to use. It would also detail if they were for resuscitation or not. Most relatives didn't wish for their relatives to be resuscitated if they went into heart failure; most wished for the most natural death possible, and most wouldn't wish to prolong their relative's illness longer than they needed to. If there were serious issues such as broken bones or severe blood loss, then this would often require hospitalisation, and usually the relatives would want some form of intervention in this instance. It was still their right to state what their wishes were for their relatives upon admission, or sometimes even before the resident's illness took hold by writing an advance directive which would state exactly the sorts of medical interventions they would wish once they had lost the capacity to state this for themselves. Any of us can write an advance directive. It has to be documented in advance of any considerable deterioration in capacity.

Once the drinks were done, this was usually the part of the day where activities with the residents would take place. There would be an activities co-ordinator some days. Unfortunately she was given the task of being in charge of all four units, so we didn't see her much. When she did arrive she would often get the residents involved in a whole manner of varying tasks, simple crafts or film afternoons. You would often find that the activities co-ordinator didn't frequent the dementia units as often as the other units.

The previous co-ordinator had left due to feeling stressed and pressurised. One co-ordinator simply wasn't going to be enough to cover up to eighty residents. The dementia units were a far bigger challenge to come up with activities and tasks that could engage. But it could be done, it just took a different approach.

The new activities co-ordinator had been given the job based on her phenomenal presentation, where she wowed the management with her big ideas and evidence based practice. What appeared a little unusual for an activities co-ordinator was that she didn't appear particularly dynamic or brimming with ideas. Most staff had discussed how she appeared very hard to speak to, and seemed to direct her orders out to everyone.

Paul had to literally drag her onto the unit one day just to talk to a new resident. She spent a total of ten minutes on the unit, and tried to introduce the resident to some painting, but he wasn't interested. She left the unit, and was not to be seen for quite some time since.

The home had recently acquired a brand new minibus, which could hold up to ten residents and carers. Most of the staff had their doubts as to its acquisition, and the rumour was that it was only bought for tax purposes. It was a blue and pink bus, and proudly displayed the company's logo all over it. Our unit had yet to utilise the bus, but we were promised that some of our residents would get full use of it during the summer months.

But there was a snag.

There would be no relatives allowed to go onto the bus. If the residents required an additional carer to go along with them, to provide assistance and support, then the relatives would get billed for the carer's hourly rate for as long as the resident was taken out for.

The activities co-ordinator had already managed to crash the minibus on one of its first outings, which had led Mick to go mad. The co-ordinator was trying to negotiate a difficult manoeuvre in a local supermarket parking space, and had managed to reverse the bus straight into another car, and dented the whole rear of the bus, causing over £500 worth of damage. There was a nurse in the passenger side of the bus, and to stop himself laughing so much, he had to quickly offer to step out for a short while and get some money out from a cash point. The co-ordinator hadn't got off to the best of starts, but it was early days yet. After this incident, a memo went round detailing that anyone who wished to drive any company vehicle would now be liable for the first £250 if they caused any damage.

I used to get involved in activities during my time as a student and people could often dismiss people with mental health issues as having sub normal levels of intelligence. I couldn't count the number of times I got well and truly beaten at draughts by some patients. On one of my placement areas the games would often be legendary and go on for several hours. By the end of the placement, several other patients would gather round and watch intently as the game progressed. I was up against an elderly farmer. He was suffering with depression and psychosis and paranoid delusional thoughts, but he could play a mean game of draughts. Every single time, I was wiped out. To this day I will always remember that as a warning beacon, to remind myself that patients should never be treated as sub standard or 'beneath us'.

I found myself holding on to these good memories of my time as a student nurse. It was often quite a crushing and difficult period of my life, but I had to hold on to the good times, and the good experiences that had helped shape me into the person I am now.

Paul looks up from his desk and turns towards me.

'I tell you what, it's been a busy day so far hasn't it?'

'Sure has,' I say.

'I'll go check on Edward soon, see if they need anything. It's a good job we have enough staff on today.'

Sharon shouts over to Paul.

'Okay if we go on a break now is it Paul?

Paul looks up. 'Yep, fine, you and Katie are going are you?'

'Yes, going for a smoke love.'

'No problem.'

It was common courtesy for the care assistants to tell you when they were going for a break. It could be as early as 3:30 p.m. or as late as 4:40 p.m; it would just depend on the daily tasks at hand. Paul would tell me that they wouldn't always tell the nurse in charge when they were going and would just automatically leave the unit. This wasn't the best thing to do, as if there was any emergency, the nurse in charge needed to know exactly where staff were and what they were doing. I had noticed that when I was a student nurse the hospitals seemed a lot stricter, and the nurses had a lot more respect from the care assistants.

Suddenly there was a loud ringing bell. Moments later Edward's daughter came running around the corner. The next few moments seemed to happen in pure slow motion; immediately I knew something was wrong. Edward's daughter shouted out to Paul.

'Come quickly.'

Paul shot up from his seat and rushed towards Edward's daughter. I stayed fixed to my seat for a few moments, until Paul snapped me out of it by quickly shouting back out to me.

'Jack.'

I shot bolt upright, and started quickly walking towards Paul. Eventually I found myself running to the room. Paul shot into the room first, and I quickly followed in.

All Edward's family were in here. There were at least a dozen or so people. Loud sobbing and crying in every direction. Edward is on his back, and looking in considerable pain, gasping for every breath. His eyes still firmly shut, shaking profusely, and I can still hear a faint crackle in his breathing.

His daughter is standing over him, and shouting out at Paul.

'His breathing changed a few seconds ago and he looks like he is in pain.'

I noticed the wife wasn't here.

The daughter is shouting to another family member.

'Get Maggie on the phone now!'

The daughter turns to Paul. 'Maggie just stepped out for a few minutes to get some fresh air.'

Another family member is on the phone frantically trying to dial. She is crying as well.

'Get Maggie, get her now!'

Edward is looking more and more agitated. A small tear starting to run down his left cheek.

'Look he's crying oh no, God, is there anything we can do?'

Edward lurches forward and goes very rigid. He slowly rests onto his back. I cannot hear any more breathing or rattling. I cannot hear anything at all. The whole room seems to be filling with shouts and tears, but for a brief second, which seems to last for minutes, the whole room falls silent to me, complete peace and tranquillity, you could almost eat up the silence in big clumps.

Paul kept calm and spoke to the daughter.

'There's nothing we can do, he's passed on.'

The daughter screams out a shrill scream.

'Noooooooooo, Dad!!!'

Another girl in the room cries out.

'Granddad, no, grandaddddd!!!'

Paul walks over to Edward and checks his pulse. From my training a radial pulse in the wrist is not a definitive pulse to check. Paul checked the pulse in his neck, the carotid artery, and turned to the daughter.

'I'm afraid he's gone. Would you like me to give you a few moments? Take all the time you need.'

I stare back at Edward, who only this morning I had spoken to. He is now lying in his bed, perfectly still. I half expect him to sit up and speak the words' half left' one last time, but he isn't going to. Edward is dead.

I didn't know where to place my eyes. All the family were crying and some were touching Edward's face gently. I walk out of the room with Paul. I feel an immense sadness come over me. Just as we were walking down I heard the click of the door again. Paul and I both turn round. Edward's wife was walking down the corridor, very tearful. Paul has a few quiet words to her and ushers her into the room. I walk into the nursing office and sit down with Paul.

I feel myself shaking. I couldn't find any words to say to Paul so we both just sat there in silence for a few moments. It wasn't like the movies, this was real life, real families, there was no glossy ending, no slick edits or cuts, I had seen everything in its full blown glory.

Eventually Paul turned to me.

'Right mate, we need to get a few things in motion.'

There were a number of things that had to be dealt with in a death. The first thing to do was to contact the local GP and inform them of the death, and various forms had to be filled in and faxed over. There was no set amount of time families could be given, they were given as long as they needed, and for now I wasn't really focusing on anything very clearly.

It was never going to be an easy thing to deal with. Even now I was thinking how I couldn't stay in this area of work forever; it was simply too much of a reminder of our own mortality. I guess the thing we have to remember is that Edward died a relatively pain free death and everything was done to provide him with the utmost care and dedication, giving him the best quality of life in his final days.

Sharon suddenly comes walking around the corner into the office.

'Has Edward passed away?'

'Afraid so,' I say.

'Right, I'm going to go and have a word with the family then, we need to clean him up, before the body gets stiff.'

Rigor mortis can set in within about twenty minutes of someone dying. This can make it very difficult to dress someone in their clothes. The usual practice would be to clean Edward up and dress him in his best clothes, before it got too difficult to do so.

'Right,' I say.

Sharon walks back up the corridor and grabs Katie who is also just coming down the corridor.

I hear a few more clicks of the door and go to see what is going on. Edward's family are all coming towards me and they walk past me and into the quiet lounge. Paul comes out of the nursing office for a brief moment and talks to each family member individually.

'Sorry for your loss.'

Paul shakes hands with all the family members. The daughter and wife are still very tearful.

Jenny comes round the corner and offers to make everyone a cup of tea. Half of them take up the offer.

A few moments pass and Sharon comes back around the corner into the nursing office.

'Right, he's ready.'

Paul ushers me towards Edward's room again.

'Right, let's just double check everything, I mean I'm sure he is dead, but we need to properly verify it for this documentation.'

The verification of death form states that you have to make an initial check, and then check twenty minutes later to confirm that there are no vital signs.

As I walk into the room I notice that Edward's body has now gone a very dull yellow colour and he is looking a lot more gaunt than a few moments ago. Paul slowly lifts each of Edward's eyes open and shines a small pen torch into them. He is checking for any pupil dilation.

'Well, he's definitely dead.'

Edward has been dressed in his best Sunday outfit, a bright red shirt and black trousers. One of his daughters left a small flower holder which reads 'world's best dad' on it, and Edward is clutching this in his arms. I half expect Edward's eyes to snap open again.

Paul ushers me out of the room again, and we walk down the corridor. As we come round the corridor to the nursing office, Paul explains to the family that he is ready if they wish to see him again. A few volunteer, but a few stay and cry in the corner.

Edward's wife comes into the office to speak to Paul.

'Hi Paul.'

'Hi Maggie, I'm sorry for your loss, he was a cracking fella your husband; I did like old Ed.'

'Well we knew it would come to this didn't we? I'm just glad he wasn't in a lot of pain.'

'No, we got him on the syringe driver quickly and I don't think he suffered at all.'

'You have been so good to him whilst he was here, so I just wanted to thank you for everything you did for him.'

'An absolute pleasure, don't worry at all.' Paul gives Maggie a quick hug. Maggie is still a little tearful but appears to have calmed down since earlier.

'What do we do now then? Have you contacted the undertakers?'

'Yep, I'll contact them as soon as your ready to leave, and then they will get in touch with you as regards the service and what they wish to do.'

'Okay,' Maggie says. 'Well I'm just going to have one more look at him and say my goodbyes and we will be off, okay Paul?'

'Okay, no problems, just let me know if you need anything.'

'Will do, and thanks again.'

Maggie walks back around the corner to go and say her goodbyes to her husband one last time. Paul begins going through the filing cabinet looking for more documentation that needs to be filled out.

Paul turns to me.

'You okay mate?'

I pause for a brief second. 'Yeah, I'm okay.'

I wasn't sure if I was okay, but I had to be. This was a part of the job and one that was inevitable for everyone here at some point.

The rest of the family walked out of the quiet lounge and met up with the wife who had just come out of Edward's room. Paul followed them up the corridor and shook each one's hand.

'Sorry for your loss.'

This went on for about two to three minutes and then all of Edward's family left the unit very slowly. It was like time had stood still. Edward had gone. I decided I wasn't actually okay, and turned to Paul.

'I just need a few minutes if that's okay, to get off the unit, do you need me for anything at the minute?'

'No, I'm fine, yeah you take yourself off the unit, all I need to do now is fill in the rest of the LCP, contact the undertakers, then you can help me write an email to the manager and owner just to inform them of the death.'

Paul grabs the notification of death form and begins filling it in.

'Time of death, 3:40 p.m.' He starts scribbling away and signing the form.

'Okay, I'll catch you in a bit then,' I say.

I go out to the store room and grab my rucksack, and walk down the long corridor, open the door, and take in one big deep breath, and sigh to myself. I mutter quietly under my breath.

'This is a long day indeed.'

I sit in the staff room; there is no one else about. The staff room overlooks the car park. I can hear the faint sounds of a bingo game being played in another lounge area. From the staff room you can see the corner of the smoking shelter. I wonder what gossip is going on in there right now, and what decisions are being made as to how the home should be run, and how the carers are going to do it. I wonder how my reputation is going within the smoking shelter fraternity.

The door opens a crack, and one of the laundry girls pops in and says hi. She is wearing a bright green and white striped top, she must be in her mid forties, with short jet black hair. I briefly saw her this morning, pushing her trolley up and down the corridor in a cheerful yet lacklustre manner.

A lot of these girls don't want any more stress in their life, they are just happy to be doing the general washing and drying each day, and keep up with the gossip from the smoking shelter. A lot of the girls are married, with their husbands earning big salaries, so these jobs for them are just a bit of pin money to enjoy at the weekend or for the odd meal or holiday. The laundry girl is emptying the bins around me, and refilling the kitchen towels. She seems happy in her position. No one bothers her, and she can just get on with things in her own busy little fashion. She smiles at me again as she leaves the staff room, and I am again left in silence.

In the far distance I can see lots of fields. There are a few static caravans awkwardly placed there. In the distance I can see an ambulance slowly making its way around the long windy road. It turns cautiously into the car park.

4–5 p.m.

The carers start to get people ready at the table for teatime, laying out the trays ready with a few pieces of cutlery and beakers of juice. A recent management meeting had revealed lots of new initiatives in order to save money.

One of the new initiatives was to scrap the existing paper napkins which were used each mealtime for more cost effective material ones. The material napkins were white. Plain white. In the long run the idea sounded a good one, until you learn that according to the laundry girls, that everything in the home was washed at a cool wash at forty degrees. They were going to stain incredibly easy and incredibly fast. All it would take is one slip of the spoon and you would have dark red stained napkins from a slight mishap with a tomato and basil pasta bake. The idea behind the new material napkins was to raise the image of the home. The carers didn't think the image would last too long once the relatives saw the faded remains of last night's meal.

Soiled laundry, soiled with urine and faeces, was only washed at a forty degree wash. The latest rumour on these wipes was that a member of the company travelled all the way to Italy on a reconnaissance mission to source the best quality wipes, purchase them, and ship them back to the home.

The laundry girls were up in arms about the next idea that was supposed to be rolling out within the next few months. Every resident's room had a box of wipes in it, for exclusive use for personal care needs. The new plan was to have re-usable wipes, which could be washed each day and returned to the rooms. Having realised that everything was only ever washed at a cool wash, the girls thought that this was one of the stupidest ideas ever invented, plus these wipes were being used on the most sensitive of areas on a resident, each day.

The current monthly budget for the wipes across the entire home was not to exceed £300. Each box contains 1,000 wipes. Each unit would be allowed six boxes each, a total of 6,000 wipes. 6,000 wipes divided into each individual resident (20), gives you 300 wipes at your disposal, per resident, for the whole month, so that works out to roughly 10 wipes per day, per resident. An average resident will get changed / toileted up to 6 times in a day and night, leaving you on average 1.6 wipes per change. If the unit ran out of wipes, it was the nurse in charge's responsibility to ring up Mick and explain exactly why the unit had run out. The cost of a single pack of wipes containing 100 wipes is around £1.07.

The units were getting through far too many wipes each day, and the company needed a new way of being able to keep an eye on costs. This was the solution, and no one was happy. The laundry girls said the plan would soon fail once they started stacking freshly washed hygiene wipes that were stained with yesterday's remains of faeces and urine. Mick was not getting a good reputation for himself, as he was one of the engineers of this bold new plan to eradicate once only uses. The laundry girls continued to uphold his nickname of 'Mick the prick'.

The carers were considerably worried about the financial position of the company, as many more cost cutting initiatives were supposedly going to roll out within the next few months. To give you a sense of just how much things could cost in a home like this, the curtains for the entire home were rumoured to have cost £50,000, as they were all from Laura Ashley and custom made.

The next idea from the management would be to reduce the amount of staff working on the unit. The suggested minimum legal requirement for the unit was actually four staff; three carers and a nurse. This equated to one staff member for every five residents. The only trouble with this is that it included the nurse in the staffing levels. This was fine in principle, however at a moment's notice the nurse could be called upon to do a number of tasks on any given day. The nurse would help out as much as they could, with feeding and assisting in getting residents up or taking residents to the toilet. The priority was always the nursing. That's what they were paid to do. They were not paid as a carer. They did the medication, they updated the care plans. They could be on call to help when the team needed it, but that didn't mean they were available for every hour of the shift.

The carers had been in a position before where they were running on only four members of staff, and they struggled. Baths got missed, the residents didn't have much time for activities, and many just sat in their rooms, bored, because the unit was stretched. The carers were hard working, and they gave it their all every shift. A few carers had been leaving lately. They had reached the end of their tether. The weekends would run short, and sickness would be higher on weekends than in the week.

One morning there were only four members of staff on, including the nurse. Emma was on this particular shift and she threatened to leave that morning. She struggled on through with her job, with all the other carers. She had started to complain to some of the relatives on that day as to how stretched they were. Paul would often say that the best way to get things done around the home would be to go through the relatives rather than the management. They were the ones with the real power. They were the ones with their significant others being cared for, and if they didn't like the way things were being run, then they would go straight to the top, and it would cascade down.

One of the relatives had agreed to ask the owner of the home just what the staffing levels should be, as he didn't feel it was right for the carers to be pushed to their limit each and every day. Shortly afterwards, the complaint was raised, and a management meeting arranged. It was agreed that the minimum staffing levels should remain at four. That day baths couldn't be completed, and the carers simply didn't have enough time to do everything. Whilst the nurse was busy doing the medication, the carers had a three way split. Two carers could pair off and start getting people up, which left one carer on their own, which would go against the company policy of working on your own and moving residents on your own.

There were very few residents that you could safely get up on your own, and one of the carers would be forced to undertake this role, whilst waiting until the nurse was free from doing the medication round. They could only do the best they could, but a nurse's role was an incredibly busy one. All it would take was a few phone calls from relatives, a resident to fall on the floor, a resident to deteriorate quickly in presentation, and the nurse was out of the picture, for the entire day. This meant the nurse couldn't help feed either.

The management warned that any member of staff telling relatives that they were understaffed would be a sackable offence and had serious implications for breaching confidentiality about staffing ratios to the relatives.

To be a carer wasn't the greatest paid job. It was barely above minimum wage. A carer could earn anything from around £12,000 - £16,000 a year, depending on experience and qualifications. Many carers would work additional hours in other homes, and have to rely on more than one income stream. The carers were your key to a strong team, and a smooth running shift. Any cracks that started to appear here would greatly affect the running of the unit on a day to day basis. The carers were your eyes and ears, they were the ones who were seeing the residents day in day out, and they could help spot any changes in their behaviour, skin condition, or general presentation. They were effectively helping to map your residents daily, and their insight and information was vital. It was a very physical and demanding role; twelve hours on a heavy unit was incredibly draining on all aspects of the body.

For the third year in a row, the home had announced that there were to be no pay rises again. No wonder the carers were feeling so lacklustre and demotivated. All they could see around them was the home spending excessive amounts of money on items such as minibuses and a newly commissioned hedge to increase the look and feel of the home in the exterior courtyard.

Some staff did get pay rises, but only a select few. The management decided each year to send out letters to staff members they thought deserved a little extra pay award. This would only amount to a few pence more an hour, but at least it was something. It was all kept secretive, and staff were urged not to tell anyone else if they had a letter.

The phone rang. Paul walked over to the phone. It was Mick. He was returning the message I had left him earlier about the stand aid.

The stand aid was going to go back to be fixed. This could take six to eight weeks. This meant that there was only going to be one stand aid left for the entire home. For eighty residents. This would mean a lot of negotiating for usage of the stand aid throughout the working day between most of the units. If this stand aid malfunctioned for any reason, then we were going to be in some serious trouble.

'If it's not a stupid question, why can't the firm borrow another stand aid or buy one?'

Paul just laughs out loud to me.

'You have no chance mate, they won't pay for anything in this place. We have to struggle and manage with what we have until something goes wrong and then the shit will really hit the fan.'

'That's not good at all.'

'Yeah, I feel bad for telling you all this mate, you're newly qualified, you don't need to hear this from me. I've been in the business far too long, it's different for you, you have come from a different era.'

'No please, I appreciate your honesty, I'd much rather people tell me like it is, than have to find out as I go along. It's important to me.'

'Well, just tell me if you think I am going on too much, just let me know.'

'I will.'

Having no stand aid would also put considerable pressure on the carers when lifting and moving the residents. To keep calling down for the stand aid was impractical, so frequently this would now force the carers to lift residents illegally by drag lifting or moving residents from wheelchair to chair without the use of the stand aid, even though they couldn't weight bear very well. This would put more pressure on carers' backs. Without the right equipment jobs couldn't be done properly. Without a stand aid you could use a hoist instead, but there was only one hoist on the unit. Due to the pressures of the unit, it would also take a considerable amount of time to hoist every resident in and out of chairs.

'If you can find Ian, we could do with getting him in the bath today. I was reading his notes from where he was last, and they said they had great difficulty with his personal hygiene, and I don't think he has had a bath for over two weeks.'

'Okay, I'll try.'

I walk around the unit until I find Ian, sitting comfortably in a chair in the lounge area.

'Ian!'

'What?'

'Just a quick question really, would you like to have a bath this afternoon?'

'A what? A bath, no, I don't need one, I will sort that out myself when I am ready.'

'It's just I can prepare you a bath this afternoon, I thought you might like one, just to settle you in?'

'No, it's okay, I can look after myself really, I don't need one.'

'I thought you could have your hair washed too, ready and nice for when your daughters visit.'

'Well, it's not really a concern of theirs, so don't tell me about them, I am a clean man. I don't need you to tell me what I need doing.'

'Okay, well how about if I run the bath for you, and let you do everything else?'

'No.'

'Are you sure Ian?'

'Yes, I can sort it out when I want one, I don't need anyone telling me otherwise.'

'I will run one for you then?'

'No.'

Ian pauses a moment.

'Listen here, I'm getting a bit offended about all this talk of having a bath. I am a very clean gentleman, and I wash every morning, I don't need anyone telling me when to have a bath. I like you, but it's just starting to get on my nerves a little bit.'

'I'm sorry Ian, I didn't mean to offend.'

I offer an outstretched hand. Ian stares at my hand for a moment, then outstretches his, and we shake hands for a good half a minute.

'As far as I am concerned, it is all water under the bridge now, okay?'

'Yep, no problems Ian, I won't mention it again.'

'Good.'

I walk back up to Paul in the office.

'It's a no go I am afraid. I tried my best, but he was getting very agitated and a little angry, but we have sorted it out now, and he is fine about things, but he is very adamant about not having a bath, so I wouldn't approach him again today.'

'Okay mate, at least you tried, I will document that anyway, and see if one of the carers has any better luck.'

'Okay.'

Paul goes back to tapping away on the computer, heavily engrossed in the screen.

I could hear some distant shouting from further up the corridor. Faint, but still audible.

'Helllooooo.'

'Hellloooo.'

'Who's that?' I ask Paul.

'Probably Donna I would expect, she does that a lot.'

Donna had been put back on bed rest for the afternoon. This was common to relieve pressure sore areas, as twelve hours sat in one place in the lounge area would be far too long to sit in one position. You would often have to put a handful of residents back in their rooms on bed rest in the afternoons.

Donna would sometimes request to go back in her bed some afternoons, and she had considerable capacity to tell staff her wishes, and some degree of understanding of her illness. She used to work as an accident and emergency nurse in the 'good old days' of nursing. Donna had Parkinson's disease with dementia.

Donna was in her early nineties. She used to have a history of falls but is no longer mobile and requires the use of a stand aid to help transfer her from bed or chair, and a wheelchair for being transferred from her room into the lounge area. As well as her condition she also has super ventricular tachycardia, or SVT (a rapid rhythm of the heart) but currently this was managed well with her medication.

Paul had encountered a few run-ins with this particular condition in the past. One morning at precisely 8:04 a.m. as he was walking down the unit corridor he was accosted by the night nurse, who was in a bit of a panic. A few beads of sweat were running down his face, and his small wireframe round glasses were actually starting to steam a little.

He guided Paul immediately into Donna's room, where Donna was describing shooting pains, and she could actually feel her heart beating incredibly fast.

'I can feel it you know, it's definitely pulsing through me.'

Paul looked a bit panicked. The night nurse had already taken her blood pressure a few times before, and it was high.

> **Blood Pressure**
>
> 'Every blood pressure reading consists of two numbers or levels. They are shown as one number on top of the other and measured in mmHg, which means millimetres of mercury. If your reading is 120/80mmHg, you might hear your doctor or nurse saying your blood pressure is "120 over 80".'
>
> - 'The first (or top) number represents the **highest level** your blood pressure reaches when your heart beats and pumps blood into your arteries - your **systolic** blood pressure. An example might be 130mmHg.'
> - 'The second (or bottom) number represents the **lowest level** your blood pressure reaches as your heart relaxes between beats - your **diastolic** blood pressure. An example might be 75mmHg.'
>
> 'Normally your target is to have a blood pressure below 140/85mmHg. However, if you have heart or circulatory disease, including being told you have <u>coronary heart disease</u>, <u>angina</u>, <u>heart attack</u> or stroke, or have <u>diabetes</u> or kidney disease, then your blood pressure should be below 130/80mmHg.'
>
> **British Heart Foundation, (2011)**

The night nurse had measured Donna's blood pressure for the last hour and they read:

210/100......

205/111........

198/101...

Paul took Donna's blood pressure again....205/100. It wasn't going down at all. Her pulse was also through the roof at 105. Most average pulses would be around the 60-80 mark. The night nurse was an RMN. Paul was an RMN. They both looked equally blankly at each other, not entirely knowing what to do. They knew something was wrong. Donna knew something was wrong.

Whilst this was all going on, the night nurse was not in the lounge area to do the hand over. His priorities had remained with Donna. Mental health nurses didn't always have extensive general nursing knowledge, but they knew that a racing pulse and high blood pressure was not a good thing.

A good fifteen minutes had passed, and between Paul and the night nurse, they had done Donna's blood pressure at least half a dozen times. Even Donna was starting to look a little confused.

'Well, what do you think we should do?'

'Are you in any pain Donna?'

'Well, sometimes I can feel a little bit of pain in my chest, but it goes straight away. I wouldn't worry about it though, I have had this before. Last time I had it, I had to go into hospital, I hate the hospital though, they always treat you quite roughly there, I don't think they understand.'

After much staring at each other and many more blood pressure readings being taken, Paul and the night nurse decided to walk back down to the nursing office and ring the out of hours doctor, and explain the situation.

The carers were still sat patiently in the lounge area, waiting for the morning handover. One of the carers had started to get a little restless. One carer walked up to the nursing station.

'So, are we getting the handover this morning then or what?'

Paul never said anything at the time, but he was silently seething. He was trying to sort out a potentially life threatening situation, a situation which was becoming more and more stressful, and all the carer wished to know is if they were going to get a handover.

Donna would often be able to describe her condition well, and how it affected her on a day to day basis. She would sometimes notably shake, particularly her hands, and refer to her illness as 'Mr Parkinson'. She would often state that 'no two days are the same'. And she would often have incredible clarity in her thinking, but other days she would have great difficulty searching for certain words, and get agitated when she couldn't come up with them. Her mood would often fluctuate.

I walk up the corridor to Donna's room. She is sat up in bed, with an assortment of toiletries strewn out all over her bed, a toiletry bag, and a large pack of biscuits by her side. She looks very pale and gaunt. She has a kind face, full of years of wisdom, with long dark grey hair.

'Helllooo!'

Donna would often shout out hello at the top of her voice, in a very shrill tone. As well as her normal Parkinson medication, she was also prescribed a Rivastigmine patch, used for mild to moderate dementia, and also known as an Acetyl cholinesterase inhibiting drug.

> **Acetyl cholinesterase inhibiting drugs**
>
> 'Acetyl cholinesterase is an enzyme which breaks down the neurotransmitter acetylcholine. Acetylcholine sends messages between nerves, signalling muscle contractions.' (Waugh & Grant, 2004).
>
> 'Rivastigmine works by increasing the concentration of acetylcholine at sites of neurotransmission (NICE, 2010). However Rivastigmine has not been studied against alternative treatments.'
>
> 'There is no evidence that Rivastigmine provides added efficacy or side effect advantages over other drugs in the same class (Ministry of Health and Long Term Care, 2009), however it has shown larger treatment benefits versus placebo in dementia with Parkinson's disease (Cummings, et al, 2010).'

Like all drugs for dementia, they are essentially used to slow down the progression of the disease, and improve quality of life for a longer period of time. It will keep people like Donna functioning at her highest level for as long as possible. It is vital that people are given this drug on a daily basis. If the medication was missed, this could potentially cause a drop in their presentation, memory, and general functioning, which would be irreversible.

They would often go out of stock. Over the past year, they have run out of stock at least half a dozen times. Most drugs are often kept in good supply, but the supplier of Rivastigmine has had particular problems at times getting its product to the home and other homes within the area. They also make the drug in tablet form, but this is not always as effective, as the elderly don't always take well to taking their tablets, and a patch is less intrusive, and will be applied on a daily basis to their back or shoulders, and alternated.

Paul had spoken to the doctor about this numerous times. They would simply state that there was a massive shortage, and they were trying their best to get hold of it, but they couldn't promise anything. We would frequently run out of stock of the drug for a few weeks at a time, causing massive problems within the home, due to the drug's importance.

The doctors' theory was that the manufacturers were simply trying to source cheaper ways and materials in which to make the drug. Staff would often wonder what went on in the higher echelons of the big and powerful corporate world of drug manufacturing.

'Donna? What's the matter?'

'Oh I'm so glad you're here, I want you to do something for me.'

'What can I do for you?'

Donna points towards her wardrobe.

'You see, in there, should be some pink slippers, can you get them for me please?'

I open the wardrobe door, and grab the small pink slippers that are hiding in the far reaches of the bottom of the wardrobe.

'These?'

'Yes, those, that's what I'm looking for, can you just place them on the bed for me please?'

'Sure, here you are.'

I place the slippers at the foot of the bed.

'Thank you so much, that's all I wanted, they're my special shoes you know, and I just wanted them close to me, so I can keep an eye on them.'

Donna would often come out with bizarre speech patterns and thought processes. This was often an indicator that she had a urine infection (commonly known in the business as a UTI, or urinary tract infection). Symptoms such as these could be very common, you would often test someone's urine to find out if there was an underlying infection. This wouldn't always be the case, but when you knew a resident well, and they started acting a little 'out of sorts', then this would usually be a good time to test things like urine. With dementia it could be tricky. People's thoughts were often confused, and it is hard to describe how you can tell someone being more confused than normal, but it happened, and it could take years of experience, and knowing your residents well.

Donna had been here in this home for a few years. She had always wanted to know what was wrong with her, as soon as she started having difficulties with her memory. Having a diagnosis can help people come to terms with what is going on, whereas other people don't want to know. When Donna was first told of her diagnosis she said she was quite upset and had a sense of dread. Whilst initially saddened by her diagnosis, she was grateful to be told, and would rather know of her diagnosis than it being kept from her.

I decided to stay and talk to Donna for a while. This was often the most powerful and rewarding thing you could do for people with dementia. We all need regular, every day, one to one social interaction, especially the residents here on this unit. Even if a resident can no longer speak, they will often retain an emotional memory, and just spending a few moments each day with them can make a huge difference.

Donna had been worried lately. She was worried she had to leave this home. Her continuing healthcare had recently been stopped.

Continuing healthcare

'NHS continuing healthcare is a package of continuing care provided outside hospital, arranged and funded solely by the NHS, for people with ongoing healthcare needs.'

'If eligible, you can receive NHS continuing healthcare in any setting, for example:

- in your own home: the NHS will pay for healthcare, such as services from a community nurse or specialist therapist, and personal care, such as help with bathing, dressing and laundry.

- In a care home: as well as healthcare and personal care, the NHS will pay for your care home fees, including board and accommodation.'

> 'NHS continuing healthcare is free, unlike social and community care services provided by local authorities for which a charge may be made, depending on your income and savings.'
>
> 'To be eligible for NHS continuing healthcare, your main or primary need for care must relate to your health.'
>
> 'For example, people who are eligible are likely to:
>
> - have a complex medical condition that requires a lot of care and support.
> - need highly specialised nursing support.'
>
> 'Someone nearing the end of their life is also likely to be eligible if they have a condition that is rapidly getting worse and may be terminal.'
>
> 'Eligibility for NHS continuing healthcare does not depend on:
>
> - a specific health condition, illness or diagnosis
> - who provides the care, or
> - where the care is provided
>
> Eligibility for NHS continuing healthcare is reviewed regularly. If the care needs to change, the funding arrangements may also change.'
>
> **NHS Choices, (2011)**

If a resident is requiring constant input, and requiring a whole host of anti-psychotic medication to manage agitation and aggressiveness then funding would usually be in place. The forms required to be filled in would be filled with technical jargon, and cover a whole host of different areas of care. Many relatives would often try to appeal the funding if it was going to be stopped. Without it, this would mean that they had to start funding care themselves. This is exactly what was going to be happening with Donna and her son.

Donna's son lived far away, but he often tried to visit, at least two to three times a week. He had power of attorney over Donna's money. Donna also had a house she still owned, which was sitting vacant, and was owned outright. Donna had assets which would have to be sold and realised as capital if she was to stay in this home. Donna's son didn't like this idea, and had already started to make arrangements, looking at other homes in the nearby vicinity which were cheaper.

Lasting Power of Attorney

'A Lasting Power of Attorney can help you plan how your health, wellbeing and financial affairs will be looked after. It allows you to plan in advance:

- the decisions you want to be made on your behalf if you lose the capacity to make them yourself.
- the people you want to make these decisions.
- how you want the people to make these decisions.'

'Having a Lasting Power of Attorney is a safe way of maintaining control over decisions made for you because:

- it has to be registered with the Office of the Public Guardian before it can be used.
- you choose someone to provide a 'certificate',

> - which means they confirm that you understand the significance and purpose of what you're agreeing to.
> - you can choose who gets told about your Lasting Power of Attorney when it is registered (so they have an opportunity to raise concerns).
> - your signature and the signatures of your chosen attorneys must be witnessed.
> - your attorney(s) must follow the Code of Practice of the Mental Capacity Act 2005 and act in your best interests.'
>
> **Directgov, (2011)**

The son had found somewhere that was around three hundred pounds cheaper a week than this home. He had already been to visit the home in question and liked what he saw. He promptly visited Donna and told her that she would have to be moved into this cheaper home, as he didn't have enough money to afford to keep her here.

Donna was extremely upset about the news, and it had made her quite tearful. She had been extremely low in mood since the visit, and had told all the members of staff that she would be leaving soon.

At the next ward round, Dr. Edwin had instructed Paul to get an advocacy service involved. This was an impartial group which could work on behalf of Donna and ask her if she really did want to leave or not. It was Donna's money, and her son had no right to move her out of the home for his own personal financial gain. Having a lasting power of attorney meant he had to be using her money for her best interests.

Once the advocacy service had been contacted, Paul waited a week, and eventually someone came to speak to Donna. He did not need very long at all; in fact Donna remained worried that she would have to leave the home, and stated quite clearly to the advocate that she wanted to 'stay here' and not to 'make her leave'.

The advocate clearly explained that whilst her son did have control over her money, it was still her money, and if she wanted to stay at this home, then she was perfectly entitled to. Donna was relieved. The advocate went to file a report. The son was not going to be happy about this intervention. He rang Paul up that same afternoon.

Whilst he had no problem with Donna's care, it was clear when he spoke to Paul that he was financially motivated, and quite upset about the decision about bringing an advocate along. He saw this as blocking his mother from being able to move homes. Paul had to explain that as a nurse we had to document and show that we are always acting in Donna's best interests.

The son didn't want to sell his mother's house, he wanted to refurbish it, and eventually rent it out. If she stayed in this home, he would not be able to afford to keep the house and would have to sell it, to help fund Donna's care. He was appalled at the high cost of the home, and whilst he was trying to appeal the funding, he felt that *he* was rapidly losing over eight hundred pounds each and every week.

Many residents would have to end up selling their home, and use their assets towards their eventual care. The fact remains that Donna still has considerable assets, and now her funding had been stopped, her assets would have to be realised. It remained her choice where she wanted to stay.

'How have you been today then Donna?'

Donna turns to me and scowls.

'Oh well, like this really.'

Donna laughs, more of a cackle than a laugh; she is very chesty.

'There is something about you.'

'What's that?'

'I cannot quite place it, but you are definitely...hmmmm. I cannot quite place it you know.'

'Well I am just me as far as I can tell.'

Donna laughs again.

'You are so brown though, I cannot understand why you are so brown, that must be out of a bottle.'

I decide to change the subject.

'Can you tell me what it was like working as a nurse?'

Donnas eyes light up.

'Oh, I could tell you everything you wanted to know, everything, those were the days, are you interested?'

'Oh yes, totally!'

'You're new aren't you? You must try to work well in this job, and it will reward you. You are at the start of your career. You keep it up, and you keep studying, and I think you will go far you know.'

'Really?'

'Oh yes, absolutely.'

Donna starts to shake uncontrollably. She tightens her face up, and shakes her fist in the air.

'Oh I hate this disease, it's such...it's such an insidious disease.'

Donna appeared to have a great insight into her illness.

'Well, I was a nurse you know, in accident and emergency. I tell you, times were different back then.'

'How were they different?'

'Well, where would you like me to start!'

Donna laughs.

'Try to start at the beginning!'

'Well, you couldn't get up to mischief in those days I tell you. I remember her name clearly; Sister Kay, she would look you up and down each morning, and check your uniform was in absolutely immaculate condition. I had to iron it each morning, and my hat, for fear of the sister telling you off and giving you punishments if she found a single crease in your tunic.'

Donna appeared to relish describing her past to me.

'You know there was a patch of grass outside the hospital that you were forbidden to cross? I didn't try to walk across it, but I know other people who did, and when they got caught, they faced the wrath of Sister Kay. They were often made to do menial tasks throughout the day, the most horrible tasks you could think of.'

I thought back to some of the horrible tasks I had been given on my last placement area by Nurse Linda. She had made me change someone's colostomy bag with some glee. I shuddered at the thought of it.

Donna continued to tell me all about her nursing days. It was fascinating to hear her describe the conditions that she used to work in.

'You keep up with your studies, that's my advice to you my young man, and you could go right to the top you know.'

'Well thank you Donna, I will certainly try.'

'You do that. You don't want to remain in here like me though, I'm no good any more, I feel old and decrepit, with this horrible Parkinson's.'

'You're not at all Donna, don't think like that. I'm here. We're all here to help you, and make sure you are looked after.'

'Oh I know, and everyone here is good, well, most of them.'

She chuckles to herself.

'But don't you worry about me, I've had my life you know.'

'You still have a life Donna, and I will be here now to talk to you every shift.'

Donna's eyes brighten.

'Will you?'

'Of course.'

'Really?'

'I wouldn't lie to you Donna.'

'Oh marvellous. I like talking to people, you know. It is no good sitting here in my room all this time is it? Now you could do something for me again, actually.'

She beckons me to sit closer still to her.

'I've got some chocolates in my wardrobe, can you get them for me please?'

I search in Donna's wardrobe, and find a huge box of chocolates, in the corner. I place them on Donna's table in front of her.

'Super, that's what I like, please take one.'

'Oh I'm okay, honestly, which one would you like?'

I open the box of chocolates, and tilt the box up slightly so that Donna can have a better look at the chocolates on offer to her. She takes a small chocolate and pops it into her mouth.

'Now then, there is one more thing I need help with.'

Donna is whispering at a barely audible level.

'Please come closer.'

I am sat right up close to Donna, there is barely a few millimetres between our faces. She looks me square in the eyes, and whispers again.

'Now then...'

I wait expectantly.

'You know what I really need.'

I pause a few more seconds.

'I really must open my bowels, can you help?'

5–6 p.m.

The tea time trolley was due any moment. The kitchen orderly on shift would bring it up and it would rattle away as it came down the unit corridor. There was usually a small lull of five or ten minutes, which allowed the carers to quickly catch their breath and wait for the impending arrival.

Most of the residents were sat at the table; a few were in the lounge chairs, sleeping. Drinks had been distributed to all, and the carers had wrapped their white plastic aprons around themselves and were sat in some of the lounge chairs waiting patiently.

I went to see how Paul was getting on. He was fumbling around in the medication cupboard, cursing under his breath. He was about to start the teatime medication round. Usually around 5:30 p.m. – 6 p.m. the medication round would start.

'I don't believe this, everything in here is practically out of date!'

Upon opening, the cupboard revealed an incredible amount of tiny white boxes all stacked neatly on independent shelves. Every month a new supply of medication would arrive for all the residents in the home, replacing what was available in the cupboard. In theory all these older medications should have been destroyed, as it was not good practice to keep medications that were out of date, or keep more medication than you needed.

As the months went on, more and more medication kept piling up in the cupboard space. There could be many reasons why the medication would get stockpiled like this. Sometimes residents wouldn't take their medication. The tablets would usually get destroyed straight away. A resident may be sleeping, so therefore unable to be given medication, so the tablets would not be popped out of the blister pack, or taken out of their boxes. This could add up as the days and weeks went on. There were twenty residents on this unit; only a few tablets would need to be missed for them to add up to a lot in the long term. Medication wastage was common, and costly.

The tablets were never usually destroyed until many months later. Whilst it was true that the management didn't like to waste things, it was also true that there wasn't normally much time in the day to actually get around to it, as it would require another nurse to counter sign the documentation to destroy the drugs. Paul had found paracetamol in the past that had been out of date for over two years.

The Care Quality Commission is a non departmental public body of the United Kingdom Government. It came about in 2009, and its sole purpose is to regulate and inspect health and social care services in England. This can include services provided by the NHS, local authorities, voluntary organisations, and private companies and care homes. Its purpose is simple: to protect the interests of people whose rights have been restricted. The last spot check the home had experienced was a few years ago, so there may well be one sometime soon.

On the last check the home passed with flying colours. Upon reading the report further, it would appear that they based the report on conversations with people at the home. It is quite interesting to note just how many awards the home has won over the past few years and how different it seems to be when speaking to the people on the 'shop floor', such as the carers, who work here day in, day out. They seem to paint a very different picture to what is being said on a daily basis.

When checks happened they appeared to talk to the right people, mainly management and a few relatives. The owner of the home was actually the chair for many of the organisations giving the actual awards.

Each resident had their own bed. Some of these beds would have cot sides, which were utilised to protect the resident from falling out of bed at night. These consisted of a wooden slat each side of the bed which pushed up and clicked into place, ensuring the resident was safe. Most of the mattresses that the residents were using were not large enough to cover the entire bed, and still left a few gaps in between the cot sides, so that a resident, could potentially have their foot or their arm trapped in between the gap. There were a few instances where a resident's hand had been trapped in between this gap, and they had subsequently had to go to hospital and have their hand x-rayed.

Before Angela had been given the sack, she had mentioned this to the managers numerous times, but no one had seemed to be interested in fixing the problem or doing anything about it.

The phone rang. Paul picked it up.

'Okay.'

He put the phone down.

'The undertakers are here for Edward, can you grab the carers and shut the doors to the people that are in their rooms please?'

It wouldn't be particularly good practice to leave all the doors open to the residents' rooms when the undertakers came walking in with a stretcher and a body bag. No one wants to be reminded of their impending demise, no matter how old they are.

I quickly walked up the corridor and started shutting some of the residents' doors in preparation. They clicked shut with a loud bang. A few moments later and the undertakers arrived, in immaculately cut black suits. Paul directed the two gentlemen to Edward's room. They were wheeling a stretcher in, and had a large plastic black bag which was sitting on top of it. They walk into the room, and Paul leaves them to it, handing them a form as he leaves. The undertakers simply nod, and get to work in transporting Edward's body to the chapel of rest, ready for funeral arrangements, and eventual cremation.

If a body is going to be cremated an additional requirement occurs. A doctor (not the home's regular doctor) will have to ring the unit, and ask the nurse in charge, if he or she thought there was any malpractice going on with the resident's death, or if they had any concerns. This is simply a check that everything was above board with the death. This occurs with cremation only, because if anything untoward was suspected, then there couldn't be an autopsy done on the body, due to the body being ash.

You would always appear to get a group of three people dying within quick succession of one another. And then months and months would go by, with no one dying. There would be particular clumps of activity in deaths. There were quiet months, and then all of a sudden within a couple of months, three residents would seem to die in quick succession.

More residents die on a weekend, rather than a weekday. Some residents would wait till their relatives were by their side, others would wait till their relatives had left them. One resident held on for an entire week with both his sons by his side, then as soon as the sons had to leave, and were walking across the car park, he drew his last breath. Death was very variable.

Relatives always wanted to know 'how long', but you couldn't say, no one could. It was impossible to predict.

Paul starts to wheel his medication trolley out into the corridor once again, for the last time today. He opens it up slowly, and starts to get out some of the medication ready. He is still whistling away to himself.

Deirdre assumes her position by Paul's side, ready and waiting to wash up the medication pots, as Paul uses them one by one. She would use the opportunity to make small talk with the nurses and carers. She had ultimate devotion for her husband Mark, never missing a day for over two years. She knew Mark was dying, but enjoyed visiting and helping out as best she could, wanting to feel useful. This was a common trait amongst some of the relatives. You would often find that some relatives would like to still hold onto that usefulness. Some would ask for their relative's jumpers to be kept to one side, in individual laundry baskets, to take each day and wash themselves, so they could still feel that they were doing something towards looking after them.

Katie comes walking up to me and takes me by the arm.

'I need some help with Daniel please.'

I walk back into the lounge area. There in the middle of the lounge area, in full view of everyone, including the very happy looking Jilly, Elsie, and Mindy, was Daniel.

Daniel had managed to get his socks off, most of his trousers, and his pants. His pad was strewn on the floor, and his legs were raised up in a cross legged fashion, giving the three ladies their own private show of Daniel's lower half. Jilly was talking to Elsie and Mindy.

'Look, that chap is on the floor there, showing everything!'

Donna was laughing to herself.

'I know, he does that a lot you know.'

She turns to Daniel.

'Daniel, whatever are you doing down there on the floor?'

Daniel looks up, still with his legs in mid air. He is a little confused at the question.

'Well I...err. I don't know really.'

I walk over to Daniel and Katie crouches down beside him.

'Daniel, can we just help you up, you're giving these ladies quite a show down here!'

'All right then.'

I crouch down, and between us, we help Daniel back up to his feet, and put everything back in place, so he is more respectable. We help to sit him gently back down on the chair. The three ladies are still chuckling away to themselves and marvelling at Daniel's display.

'Are you okay there ladies?'

'Oh yes, it's not often you get a little show in the evening now is it!'

'Certainly not, I think Daniel was just a little confused.'

'Well, we often see him on the floor, but not quite like that!'

All three ladies laughed together.

Lack of time is one of *the* major complaints from the nurses, across all the specialities. One of the leading works on this is the Tidal model. The tidal model specifically covers nursing perceptions of time, and how they feel a distinct lack of it. In the model it argues that this perceived lack of time to talk to residents is more about the institution itself, and its constructed nature of the 'nurse – patient relationship' itself, within 'the system'. It suggests it is how nurses conceptualise mental health problems themselves, rather than the actual time available to nurses each shift.

The old classic reason still maintained was that nurses were simply 'too busy doing other things' to talk to their patients, or engage with them therapeutically on any regular or structured basis. The evidence suggests that residents are *more* likely to act out in destructive ways the less time a nurse spends with them. What happens next is the nurse then has to become increasingly focused on suppressing these destructive ways and attention seeking behaviour in order to keep the unit or ward safe, usually with as required medication.

The Tidal Model

The most common reasons listed in the tidal model, that nurses give for not having time to spend with their residents:

- 'Too busy - keeping the ward safe'
- 'Too busy - fire fighting and crisis management'
- Too busy doing one to one observations or 'sitting on the door'
- 'Too busy doing paper work and administration'
- 'Too busy on the phone in the office'
- 'Too busy being available to medics 'on demand'

Barker, (2001)

This is part of the reason that most nurses end up getting constantly stressed, and potentially placed at risk with volatile residents. This in turn causes the residents to see their experiences as distinctly non therapeutic. A vicious circle thus ensues. Never underestimate the value of one to one time with residents, no matter how little time you can offer. It goes a long way.

I could hear the faint clattering of the tea trolley coming down the corridor. It was wheeled accurately into place, and Katie begins getting her bowls ready. Whoever was in charge of the meals liked to operate in a slightly different way from the others. They liked things their way; if the other carers tried to help out, then sometimes they could get into heated arguments.

Some would like to write down exactly which residents were in their rooms, and who was in the lounge area. Some would split the diabetics into a separate list, and then you had residents who were on pureed foods. Everyone's method was slightly different, but they all worked, efficiently and effectively.

'What have we got today then Katie?'

Katie begins taking out the large silver square pans of food, and opening them up one by one. Vast amounts of steam rise out of each one. The food would often be piping hot, sometimes too hot to initially give to the residents.

'Hmm, looks like beans on toast tonight!''

'Beans on toast!' Sharon shouts out.

'It's getting worse isn't it! Well have we got the toast then?'

'No, we have the bread though, I'd get toasting if I were you!'

'Well the other units have the toast brought up to them you know, it's getting ridiculous this is.'

The meals would often be quite varied and nutritious, however other days they could appear more simplistic and plain. There would be a new roll out in the future. Talks had already been done, and the new company was about to roll them out in the following weeks. There had already been a taster session done, and the verdict was unanimously positive.

There would be frozen meals, shipped to the home on a weekly basis. The pureed meals would be sculpted to look like a proper meal, so the carrots, instead of being some bright orange substance, would still be a bright orange type substance, but sculpted to look like formed carrots. This would further help fuel the rumours that the company was trying to streamline itself and save more money. The meals were cheaper to produce, and would also mean that they needed less input from kitchen staff. The kitchen staff were already panicking. Whilst they liked the idea of easier mass produced meals, they also realised that this could potentially mean they were out of a job.

The company assured them that they were only going to use this cheaper and quicker option to cover kitchen staff holidays. The verdict was still out, and tongues were already wagging. If you could wholesale in pre frozen ready-made meals which required no preparation, except for heating them up each day, and it was cheaper, more time efficient, then I'm suspecting that you wouldn't need so many staff to help prepare fresh foods.

As well as beans on toast today, there were a varied selection of sandwiches, each cut into tiny triangles. A selection of both white and wholemeal bread, the sandwiches were quite inventive in their creation. Coleslaw salad, prawn mayonnaise, tuna mayonnaise, chocolate spread, lemon curd, and jam. Desert was a fine selection of cup cakes. The kitchen had recently won a five star award for its selection of food. There was a vegetable patch towards the back of the home where they were attempting to grow fresh produce. It wasn't quite ready to be rolled out at present. The meals would vary considerably on a day to day basis.

Katie was cheerfully plating up the feed meals, and she thrust one into my hand.

'Can you feed Bob please before he gets up and walks away again? He's just behind you.'

Bob was sat down in his chair with his eyes half shut. I quickly sit opposite him and start to feed him.

'Hi Bob, I've got your tea here for you, some lovely soup.'

Bob doesn't respond. I begin gently spooning the food into his mouth. His eyes are still half shut. He seemed to still want his tea though, and to enjoy it. Bob would frequently be able to eat whole dinners with his eyes shut. He would often walk up and down the unit for hours on end. He was starting to get a little restless in front of me, and stood bolt upright all of a sudden. He paused a few seconds, stood up, then sat back down again, and I continued spooning his soup into his mouth.

Mindy is sat on the far table, staring miserably at her beans on toast. She tries to wave her hand and get the attention of one of the carers. Sharon looks up at Mindy.

'I don't like this, it tastes horrible.'

'I don't blame you love, would you like some sandwiches?'

Mindy doesn't appear to have heard correctly, but Sharon quickly removes her plate of beans, and puts a plate of sandwiches down in front of her.

'Right, thank you.' She half smiles as she stares down at her assortment of sandwiches.

A few short moments pass and Mindy suddenly stands up and shouts out.

'Can I go to the toilet please?'

Mindy always asked to go to the toilet, right in the middle of tea. She knew where the toilet was, and was quite able to attend to her own personal hygiene, but would always ask permission. She walks over to the window and outstretches a hand and calls to Paul who is still doing the medication.

'Miss, take me to the toilet please.'

'Ah Mrs Goggins! How the devil are you?!'

Mindy doesn't understand what Paul has said, but Paul gently offers a hand, and walks her a few paces past the open window.

'Right ,I'm okay now thank you, will you wait for me?'

'Yes Mrs Goggins, no problems, I will be here!'

Mindy walks off and around the corner to the toilet.

A few moments later Mindy returns, and Paul repeats the whole process in reverse, guiding her back into the lounge area. Paul is merrily dispensing tablets one by one. Once a few empty pots stack up on his medication trolley, Deirdre quickly whips them away and starts washing them up in the kitchen sink in the lounge area.

Paul prepares another few pills and starts walking towards Mindy. She has sat back down in the lounge.

'Hello Mindy, I've got your tablets for you!'

Paul confidently holds a small plastic pot of tablets up in his hand, with another pot filled with water. Mindy looks at Paul quizzically.

'I've had those already!'

Paul shakes his head.

'These are your tea time tablets.' Paul tries to talk as slowly as possible, as clearly and loudly as he can.

'No, I've had them, how many?'

Paul moved the pot into Mindy's direction so she could clearly see the three round tablets in the bottom of the pot.

'Three?'

'Yes, three.'

'No I'm not taking them, who told you I had to have them?'

'The doctor.'

'What for?'

Paul taps his hand on his chest, and mouths the word at the same time,

'Chest.'

'No, my chest is fine, I'm not taking them any more, you can tell him from me.'

Paul decides to go and get the whiteboard, and write down clearly in bright green pen two words: 'diabetes', and 'chest'. He walks back over to Mindy and shows the whiteboard too her, so she can clearly read the words on the board.

She looks a little confused.

'No, I've had them, my chest is fine.'

Paul motions again with the pot in his hand, eagerly waving it in front of Mindy.

Mindy's body language starts to change drastically. She scowls, and her cheeks start to redden.

'No I'm not having them I told you, you can bloody take them back with you.'

Paul gently gestures the pot in front of Mindy's face.

'No.'

And again.

'No.'

Paul had, for this evening anyway, decided that this was long enough, and he was not going to push things any further. The irony being that Mindy's third white tablet was Olanzapine, an anti-psychotic medication, that could have helped calm her down a little more.

'No, take them away will you, I am not having them!'

Paul takes the pots away from Mindy, and walks back to his medication trolley. As he passes me he casts me a knowing smile.

'I'll mark that down as a refusal then shall I?!'

Paul's next task was to give Lucy her medication. You would only have a specific window of being able to give her medication out. Usually one attempt was all you got. Her mouth would open, and that would be it. After that, it would clamp shut for the rest of the evening, and nothing you said or did would allow her mouth to open again. It was incredibly fine tuned, and Paul had learnt the art of it, over a great deal of time.

He walks up to Lucy, who was sat with her bright blue bib on, still tapping her feet on the floor.

'Hello Lucy!' Paul bellows out.

'Hello.'

'I've just got your tablets for you.'

'All right.'

'Open up then.'

Paul gradually eases the spoon towards Lucy's mouth. He just touches the plastic spoon against her slightly moist lips, and immediately Lucy opens her mouth. Paul quickly inserts the spoon, and Lucy takes the tablet.

A few moments pass. Lucy has firmly clamped shut her mouth now. She begins chewing the tablet in her mouth, rolling it from one side to the other. A frown creeps up slowly on her forehead.

'Ohh, that's bloody horrible that!'

'Sorry Lucy, I've just got an eye drop to put in as well.'

Paul gradually takes a small eye drop canister out from his pocket, and carefully just slowly pulls down on Lucy's right eyelid a little, and gently administers an eye drop. Lucy quickly flinches a little.

'No no no no no. Horrible.'

'That's it all done now Lucy, thank you, I'll leave you alone now.'

Lucy goes back to tapping her feet gently on the lounge floor, one arm locked in place, neatly under her chin, looking inquisitively with one eye back out at everyone in the lounge area. The other eye is firmly shut.

Katie is almost half way through dishing up all the tea. She has Sharon as her 'runner', taking the meals to the residents that can eat by themselves. The rest of the team are finishing off with the feed meals.

'How we doing ladies, everything going okay?' Sharon shouts out.

'Yes, I'm quite all right thanks,' Lucy shouts.

The door on the far side of the lounge opens. A gentleman walks through, carrying a large clear plastic box of paper packages. He is dressed in an immaculate white shirt, wearing thick black wireframe glasses. He has a receding hairline. He walks confidently through the corridor, and says hello to everyone. He is bringing the medication that was ordered this morning. Sometimes extra medication would be needed, a fax would normally be sent each morning detailing exactly what was needed for each patient. If that was sent early enough, then this would normally mean that you got them delivered that evening.

The gentleman walks up to the nursing station. Paul has got his head buried in the medication trolley, desperately trying to search for some eye drops. He eventually raises his head from the trolley and greets the man. The man passes over a few packages to Paul, and Paul signs a sheet. They have a brief chat about the weather, and then the man gets ready to be on his way.

'There's no Rivastigmine patches again I'm afraid...Supplier shortage, a national shortage this time.'

6–7 p.m.

Jennifer storms past Paul and I, appearing a little flustered.

'We have to talk about something now.'

She looks around to see if anyone is in the near vicinity, notices a few relatives in the lounge area and walks into the nursing office and shuts the door firmly behind her.

'It's nothing bad...just very important.'

Paul and I sit down attentively, and quickly look at each other.

'Right. We need to discuss getting people up in the morning, and the night staff.'

I wonder what could possibly have happened to get Jennifer up here and in such a panic.

'There's a home nearby that is being investigated for institutional abuse. The CQC have got their feelers everywhere, and they are crawling all over this one with great enthusiasm. They're saying that this home is purposefully getting residents up in the morning who aren't fully awake.'

Paul and I look at each other in amazement.

'At the end of the day we can no longer have day staff putting pressure on the night staff to get more people up than they should need to. If a resident is awake at a certain time in the morning, then we get them up, but under no circumstances should we awaken our residents and get them up just to please the day staff and make their day easier. This is twenty four hour care, and we are working towards the best interests of our residents, and not the best interests of our carers.'

Paul nods his head.

'I agree with what you're saying, and whenever I have done night shifts I have felt this incredible pressure upon me from about six a.m. to start getting residents up. I never usually managed more than about five, and the carers would often scowl at me and give me a look that could kill. You are going to get an incredible amount of backlash from this if not many residents are up early in the morning.'

Jennifer tightens her face.

'Yes, I appreciate that, but all the night staff need to update everyone's night care plans. If a particular resident wakes early, or wakes later, it all needs to be documented, we need to have a rationale for every decision we make. It's all paperwork, but that is what needs to be done. It's no longer acceptable to have this pressure from day staff on the night staff to get people up. It's not acceptable to have only two members of staff getting eight or more people up in the morning, especially when they are in the last two hours of their working shift, and at their most tired.'

I sensed the day staff were going to have a field day with these new revelations. This was going to cause no end of problems and bickering between them and the night staff. A night nurse had got so fed up of being asked how many residents she had got up each morning that she had taken it upon herself to contact the NMC herself and ask for some advice.

Once a little bit of pressure is put on people they usually have to do something about it. I didn't blame the nurse at all, we were having to fight for our residents in every way possible, and do the best we could for them, but we needed the support from management and staff to be able to do this.

Paul shook his head.

'This is fine in theory, however what with taking the unit down to only four staff on a working day, then this will really start to eat into the amount of time we have to actually get the residents up of a morning. Are we really expected to be able to cope with that? What if there are only two residents up in the morning?'

'You can work around it. Not everyone has to be got up in the morning in some task based race, this is twenty four hour care and we don't have to get everyone up by eleven, we can get people up at midday, and we can certainly bath people at any time of the day.'

'Well, I hope you're ready for the backlash, that's all I can say.' Paul shakes his head.

'This isn't going to go away, we need to be doing things better, and because of this investigation, we need to make sure we change things now. It has gone on for too long; please make sure you pass this on to all the day staff here today and the night staff, and if night staff can start compiling their care plans for typical waking hours of a resident that would be great.'

'Okay, will do. This is going to throw the whole day out potentially though, the carers will not be impressed.'

'Listen, at the end of the day, the carers don't run the unit, we do, and who are we looking out for at the end of the day? We are supposed to be working for the residents' best interests, you don't have to get people all up at exactly the same time, and you can bath people in the evenings if need be. We need to act on this now. We also need to start emailing management every Friday just with a brief summary of what has happened in the week; we need to be getting more efficient in communication. It doesn't need to be much, just a summary of any agency used in the week, and if anyone has been off sick, and any incidents with residents, so if you can start that as of this Friday, then that would be great.'

Jennifer throws open the door to the nursing office, and strolls confidently out of it. Paul looks a little shell shocked.

'Well that's going to go down well in the debrief isn't it!' Paul continues to shake his head.

If the nurse in charge had time, there would usually be a debrief at the end of every shift, usually around 7:30 p.m. -7:45 p.m. Most importantly these debriefs would happen after every doctor's round to keep everyone up to date on any changes that might have occurred with some of the residents. It was always nice to touch base with the staff on the unit and ask if they had any issues or points to raise during the day. It could often turn into a moaning session, but they usually appreciated the time to air their opinions.

Institutional abuse

The subject of waking hours, and waking our residents in the morning would be an ongoing battle and topic for discussion. I never did many night shifts, but on one of the night shifts I did, my unit manager actually asked me how many people were up. I evaded the question by stating that I never counted, and it should be about the quality of care. She replied by asking me directly how many people I had personally got up.

I hadn't got anyone up. There were two carers on that night, and I had been expressly told to get my care plans up to date by the unit manager herself. There were in fact four people up that morning out of nineteen residents. My unit manager told me (and the four carers that were on that morning) that we 'had to wake people'. The carers had got up the residents that were awake that morning, everyone else had been fast asleep and settled, and their pads had been changed. The unit manager herself had been known to give residents unprescribed enemas, and re-catheterise without having formal training in this procedure. This would also be classed as a form of abuse.

'Institutional abuse is the mistreatment of people brought about by poor or inadequate care or support or systematic poor practice that affects the whole care setting. It occurs when the individual's wishes and needs are sacrificed for the smooth running of a group, service or organisation.'

'In formal settings institutional abuse is more likely to occur when there is:
- No flexibility in bed times or getting up or deliberately waking someone up.
- Strict, regimented or inflexible routines or schedules for daily activities such as meal times, bed / awakening times, bathing / washing, going to the toilet.'

Harrow Council, (2011)

In the end, the other dementia unit had put in place a new plan. They were to start their six in the morning pad checks at five am instead. This was to ensure the carers were finished by six am, and had a clear two hours to get more people up from 6 a.m. – 8 a.m. The unit manager on that unit had admitted that her 'girls were exhausted' in the morning from getting so many people up, as not enough residents were being got up by the night staff.

The residents were checked and pads changed every four hours. A check at 10 p.m., 2 a.m., and 6 a.m. Sticking to strict staffing levels would sometimes mean that the carers did have a harder morning, depending on the amount of residents up. They could only do as much as they could. It was often suggested to have more carers on in a morning to alleviate these pressures, and continue with good quality care.

The home were final on their decision, and wished to work to a strict policy of five staff members in a morning, and four in an afternoon. Night staff still felt pressurised to get people up in the morning to appease day staff.

This had been an ongoing battle with night nurses and day staff. One night nurse had even been told by the unit manager that she had been monitoring her and had discovered that she 'always got five people up in the morning'. The nurse was furious, so furious that she emailed the unit manager the very next day with the following email:

'Dear Jodie,
With further response to our recent conversation, whereby you believed me to be getting a maximum number of 5 residents up every morning and in turn stated that as my manager you were telling me to "get more residents up and dressed in the morning" and to "start at 05:30 a.m.", I wish to take this opportunity to reiterate my reasons as to why the number of residents I get up fluctuates. I have been trained and believe that the essence of nursing care for older people is about

getting to know and value people as individuals, to maintain their dignity, freedom of choice and to ensure that their informed decisions are listened to and respected.'

'I fully understand the nature of the illness and traits within dementia and therefore respect that many residents may lack the capacity to make such decisions, but also appreciate that this capacity can change frequently, therefore I ensure that each person is asked in the morning if they wish to get up or not.'

'Within the guidance of our governing body (NMC), as a professional I am personally accountable for the actions and omissions in my nursing practice and must always be able to justify any decision I make. This is the reasoning behind my varying number as I truly believe that getting a resident out of bed before they are ready and willing is abuse and when a minimum number is put on how many have to be up and dressed, I maintain that this comes under institutionalisation'

"**Institutional** – 'mistreatment of a person or persons by a regime or individual staff; it occurs when the needs of the institution are put before the needs of people in their care." (NMC, 2009)."

'I have quoted the above because of your reasoning for checking how many people I get up in a morning, that being because it took your day staff till after midday to wash 15 people. My role here is to care for the residents' needs with consideration for the staff, not vice versa.'

'On the morning you approached me I had reasons for the residents you pointed out were awake, them being one had a suspected UTI and the other made an informed decision to remain in bed, stating " I bloody

> don't want to get up, No!" We also had a resident up and awake who needed to be monitored as there are issues with him becoming inappropriate with female residents.'
>
> 'I am both passionate and honest about my nursing and will continue to give the best care I can to the residents in this home, encouraging person centred care, informed choices and respecting the decisions they make. Should day staff feel that it is in the residents' best interest to be out of bed and socialising first thing in the morning i.e. if they retired to bed early the previous day, then ultimately if this is communicated to me at hand over I will be more than happy to work to the best interest of that person as it is then my duty of care.'
>
> 'I hope this difference of opinion does not affect our working relationship, but may I please ask that in turn you respect me as a practitioner and know that throughout the night and before I leave my shift, each and every resident has been cared for on an individual basis.'
>
> The night nurse never got a response from this email. The battle continues to ensue between night and day staff.

The point raised was valid: we shouldn't be getting people up and dressed when they didn't wish to be. Paul was right though, this was going to cause a lot of stress and anger amongst the carers, who practically based their whole shift on how many people were up in a morning. There could only ever be so much time in a morning to get people up, so people would have to start being got up after lunch, and this would cause havoc with everyone's break times and general morale.

With a strong team and the right number of staff, everything could be done to the best of your ability. The unit was struggling, and staff members were feeling lacklustre and in a poor frame of mind. They were now being told they had to spread out their day and tasks, and start looking towards the person centred care approach, but with less staff.

If the night staff didn't get many people up, then the day staff would leave lots of people up at night for the night staff to put to bed. It was up to Paul to start cascading this information down this evening, and see how the carers took the news.

Sharon popped her head round the nursing office. She didn't miss a trick. She looked eager to gain information.

'Everything all right love?' she enquires of Paul.

'Yeah, fine, just a few things I need to run through, I will tell you all in a debrief this evening okay? Just let the others know I want to talk to everyone.'

'Okay love, everything all right?' You could see Sharon was desperately trying to fish for further information to take back to the 'troops'.

Paul wasn't going to budge.

'Fine, I'll tell you in a bit okay?'

'All right love.'

Sharon scurried off to the lounge area. I could hear her whispering to Emma and Katie; they were already trying to decipher exactly what the visit from Jennifer was about, and trying to work out if there was going to be bad news.

I could hear the final clattering of pots and pans from the lounge area. Tea was coming to a close, and the carers were tidying the plates up from the residents' tables. The carers began to wash and clean each of the resident's faces, and help themselves to the odd sandwich that might be left over.

Historically the owner of the home had let the carers have any leftovers after all residents had been fed at teatime. By this time in the evening, everyone was pretty tired, and feeling hungry, so they would often be very grateful of the odd snack on the go, before putting some of the residents into bed.

Around this time of day, the carers would sit down and make themselves a cup of tea. People would start to be put to bed no earlier than 6:30 p.m., so once the tea trolley had finally been loaded up with dirty dishes and cups, it was time for the nominated carer to go and make everyone's drink. There was a real sense of camaraderie at this point in the evening. The carers didn't always get on with one another, but they had to work together, for a long amount of time, so they would often put their issues on hold and joke with one another. Sharon was sat down speaking to Katie. Both were sitting down in the lounge chairs.

'You will never guess what has happened to that activities co-ordinator now!'

Katie looks intrigued.

'What now?'

'She has only gone and crashed the bus again!'

'What!'

'Seriously! Not only that, I heard she was sacked, and not coming back for good!'

'What the hell! How?'

'She was taking some residents out, and hadn't strapped one of the residents in properly. So as a result, when the bus stopped suddenly, the resident fell out and hit her head.'

'Oh my god!'

'Oh, it gets better. She helps the resident back up into her seat, and takes her back to the home. Never mentions it again. The next day the resident is feeling a little faint, and vomiting all the next day. The staff finally ask her what could have possibly caused her to vomit. The resident had enough about her to eventually explain what happened on the bus. The co-ordinator had completely covered it up, she had even asked the resident not to mention anything! Well that was all Jennifer needed. The official word is that the co-ordinator respectfully stepped down from her post. But I heard she was sacked, plain and simple.'

'Unbelievable.'

'You couldn't make this stuff up if you tried love, could you? And, get this, there is already a new activities lady that has been hired! The post never went out to tender, they just grabbed the nearest lady, who comes in a few days a week to help a few of the ladies out with some basic crafts. Jennifer handed her the job immediately!'

'Wow. I can't believe she covered that up!'

'She might have had a chance if she had just owned up, but you can't do that sort of thing and expect to get away with it can you? Oh well, we shall see what the new co-ordinator is like, hey!'

'Yeah!'

The final hurdle was in sight; only a few more hours, and the carers could relax at home, ready to do it all again the following day. There would often be some joking around as to who was going to make the drinks.

Like any workplace, there would always be some conflicts and bad feeling amongst work staff. There was a particular young carer who could cut glass with her acid tongue. Most of the carers despised her, and thought that she was trying to act a lot older than her years. Using youth on her side, she felt she could use this to her advantage and use people in any way she could. Some of the carers would stand up to her, and she would almost certainly back down, but others liked the easy life, and decided to bite their tongue when they could. This was easier said than done at times.

She had already accused two of the carers of bullying, saying that they were ordering her around. What they were actually doing was directing her to the necessary tasks of the day, with no malice or sinister undertones intended, telling her who she could feed next. This had started to bother the young upstart, and she had gone straight to the owner of the home and complained. Bullying is a serious offence, and it is also a very serious offence to accuse someone of it, so the matter had to be investigated accordingly. The two carers who were accused of being bullies were understandably heartbroken, and their morale was soon crushed when they were both sat in the manager's office, asking to explain their behaviour. They were kept under constant surveillance. Eventually the case was dropped. There was no real evidence. The two carers continued to work on at the home. It was never nice for your practice to be called into question, particularly within an environment such as this, and even more so considering they hadn't done anything wrong. They never received an apology from the upstart to this day.

The upstart would continue to carry on working at the home, but if something bothered her she would continue to go straight to the top, or mouth her opinion out loud to everyone who would listen. Jenny had fallen foul of her acid tongue in the past, when it was coming up to the end of a shift. It was 7:56 p.m. The carers had finished their shift, and were just winding down, all sat around one of the main tables in the lounge area, chatting away, and waiting for the next four minutes to pass.

The upstart had come in early, due to start a night shift, and was sitting around the table with the rest of the carers. A female resident was walking around the table, moving the odd bit of furniture, and touching the table in a feverish manner.

'I'm sure I can smell something you know.'

Jenny was tired, and took the comment lightly, and replied back that she couldn't smell anything. The upstart continued to say she could smell something. She pressed on and continued to bark out an order to Jenny.

'Well, are you going to do something about it or not?'

Jenny hadn't got the patience any more. She had worked a long hard twelve hour shift, and she was beat. She simply replied back,

'I've finished work now'.

The upstart screwed up her face in disgust.

'Well I think that's disgusting,' and walked off to the nursing station.

Jenny was sat there in disbelief. The upstart was literally about to start her shift in the next few minutes, but there she was trying to bark out an order to her to go and clean up a resident. She bit her tongue, and eventually took the female resident off to be changed. This took only a few minutes, and by the time she had changed her, it was gone eight o'clock. As Jenny began to collect her bag and her coat from the store cupboard, the upstart had sat down in the lounge area, ready for a handover from the nurse in charge. The upstart in a semi sarcastic tone shouted out:

'Thank you Jenny.'

Jenny, who normally is a mild and meek individual, took one glance back at the upstart.

'Fuck off.'

Jenny walked off the unit, her face reddening, and tears beginning to form. The upstart didn't follow her or reply to her cutting remark. Jenny had worked hard for the company, and she was starting to feel the strain a little from the upstart's remarks, not just today, but for a number of weeks now. Everyone was starting to get a little fed up. That day she just had enough, and snapped.

The upstart appeared to relish in the company's almost hourly changes during the day. She would have no problems with going straight to the manager or owner for anything. She had recently reported one of the kitchen staff for doing drugs, claiming she had seen remains of cocaine on the toilet seat. He was soon sacked, despite originally being friends with the upstart, and claiming that she had been doing drugs herself at a recent house party a few nights beforehand. Statements were produced, and he was soon out of a job. She had a husband who also worked for the company, on the same unit. They would text each other during the day, and ring to keep one another updated on any gossip or day to day run ins with other staff members.

Jenny had caught the upstart's husband walking up the stairs, on the phone to his wife, giving her a run-down of the morning's events. Jenny had enough, and wasn't feeling particularly well, when she was walking up the stairs. She grabbed the phone off the husband, and began jokingly telling his wife what she had been doing, in a very sarcastic manner.

'Hi, well I have had a coffee this morning, and then I went to the toilet, then I went to get a resident up, is that okay for you?'

The husband had looked a little shocked when Jenny passed the phone back to him. Jenny just continued to stroll confidently up the stairs and back onto the unit.

Today Sharon had been the nominated tea maker, and she was already walking off at a terrific pace towards the kitchen area.

'Right Jack and Paul, what are you having loves?'

'Tea no sugar would be great,' Paul replied.

'And you Jack?'

'Coffee, milk no sugar please.'

'Jenny?'

'I'll have my usual. Tea, two tea bags, make it strong as bull's blood, with a hint of milk please ta!'

'All right love, coming right up.'

I decided to go and sit in amongst some of the ladies at the top table. I had learnt from my university days that it was always good to try to be involved with the residents as much as I could, and not try to separate myself, creating a 'them' and 'us' scenario. Sure we were having a bit of a breather, but why not have a cup of coffee with the residents and chat with them? The same applied to when nurses were writing their daily entries in the nursing notes. Most nurses in the hospital would bury themselves away in the office, and labour away at them.

As a student I would often be allowed to make entries in the nursing notes, as long as I had them countersigned by a qualified member of staff. I would always make the effort, if it was possible, to sit out in the main lounge areas, and write notes amongst the patients. There was no real reason to sit in the office, it was just a shame no one really took the lead with writing documents in this way. There was no hard and fast rule where you had to write them. Elsie, Jilly, and Donna were at the table.

'So this is where the meeting is being held is it ladies! This must be the top table here! What have you found out, what has been discussed?'

Donna laughed profusely. Her wheezing could be heard just underneath her laughing. Quiet but raspy undertones.

'Well, we haven't really discussed anything today, except the scones of course.'

Jilly looked at me and smiled. Elsie was also smiling, but her hearing wasn't as good as the other ladies, so she had to take comfort in observing body language and some of the other ladies' reactions.

Jenny shouts over to me.

'Hey, switch the stereo on behind you please Jack, let's make it a bit more lively!'

I glance behind me and switch on a large multi disc stereo. It whirs into gear and loudly booms out Max Bygraves' version of 'Kiss me goodnight Sergeant Major'. Donna's eyes immediately light up and she starts singing along. I remember I have some recent pictures on my phone, from a trip to Alicante last summer.

'Hey, would anyone like to see some pictures of my holiday in Spain?' I enquire.

Donna's face immediately lights up.

'Spain! Ooh yes, I would, let's see some pictures.'

I get my phone out and begin flipping through some pictures of the holiday, showing shots of the aeroplane cruising over parts of Spain, the hotel pool, and some random shots of the beach. Donna is genuinely showing signs of interest.

I show Elsie and Jilly the pictures in turn. Jilly turns to me.

'I can't see it love, my eyes aren't so good I'm afraid, did you have a nice time though?'

'Oh yes, a good time, it was nice.'

'You are lovely and brown though, I swear that must be out of a bottle though?'

'No, it's real!' I laugh.

'It's just I really don't understand how brown you can be, it's incredible!'

Elsie turns to me.

'Did you fly over the Alps then if you went to Spain?'

'I sure did!'

I quickly find a shot out of the plane, cruising over the Alps. Elsie's eyes light up.

'I went to Spain, years ago, twice in fact. My memory isn't that bad you know! I'm not dementing just yet!'

Her memory wasn't fading just yet, and she would remember a lot. In this line of work it would be so easy to pigeon hole people as having a completely failed memory, unable to do anything for themselves. This was often not the case.

Everyone was different, and had different stages of dementia. Everyone was an individual and had to be treated as such. Elsie could remember your name, and have a sense of you not being there for a particular period of time. Other residents may also have that sense, but not be able to vocalise it, which would be a more emotional memory, but it would still be there.

'I was on a gondola once you know! Being serenaded to! In Venice, I'm talking a long time ago now! Must be at least forty years!'

She smiled, and as she smiled I saw a hint of sadness in her smile.

Jilly asked me who was on tomorrow.

'It's me again, and Paul tomorrow.'

'Oh is it! Are you sure?!'

'Yes, it's definitely us two tomorrow.'

'I like Paul, he makes me laugh, he calls Mindy Mrs Goggins, but she doesn't know that as she's deaf, and he's always telling me that I'm laying eggs because I sit on my chair for a long time in the day!'

Paul could inject humour into the day, and in a job like this, it was paramount to get back to the residents' sense of humour, if only for a few moments. It was worth its weight in gold. Paul had a real knack for it, and the years of experience really showed. He was able to crack jokes in a split second, and really make the residents smile. At times you would think how futile everything was, as this was the residents' final resting place, but they were still alive, they still had a lot to offer.

As mental health nurses we were there to help guide and bring that out in them, give them the best life we could, and try to let them enjoy every day. It was a real skill, that insidiously massages itself throughout the working day, not always able to be written down and not always able to be taught in the traditional sense in a lecture theatre.

You can read the theory day in, day out, and be the best theorist and activist of the literature. But sometimes you just had to go with your gut feeling, and instinct, when speaking to people. Sometimes life just kind of happens, and you go with the flow. You adapt, roll with it.

I carried on chatting to the ladies. I thanked them for their time, and said I would be back shortly to help them get ready for bed, or move them into the lounge area to a more comfortable seat. As I got up to walk into the kitchen I heard Jilly talking to Donna.

'He's a nice lad isn't he!'

'Oh yes, a really nice lad, I think we will keep him you know.'

A few moments passed. I was having a contemplative moment over the day's events, when all of a sudden a gentleman came into view in the doorway to the office. He was fairly short, with an intense stare, and greying hair. He had a look of mild worry on his face, as his forehead wrinkled up a little as he spoke. Gerry Wilkins, son to Graham Wilkins, his father had been on the unit for a good number of years.

'Paul, I think you had better come see this'.

Paul leapt up from his chair, and followed Gerry to his father's room. I wasn't sure whether to follow or not.

A few moments passed, and Paul came rushing back into the nursing office. He didn't speak to me, but quickly went to grab the blood pressure machine.

Before I could shout to Paul if he needed any help, he was gone. Another few moments passed, and he came back into the nursing office, looking a little red around the cheeks. He shouted to the rest of the carers.

'Has anyone emptied Graham's catheter bag today ladies?'

Sharon, Katie, and Emma, all looked at one another, and all shook their heads solemnly.

'No, not today.' Paul turns to me.

'Right mate, another problem to sort, can you get one of the carers to help you? We need Graham on his bed and on his back, I think he's gone into retention.'

Urinary retention is a lack of ability to urinate, usually a lack of output or an intermittent flow. Sudden onset of retention can be very serious, and could require hospital admission. If the bladder continues to remain full it can lead to a whole host of other more serious complications, increasing pressure and in some cases it can cause urine to pass back up the ureters and get into the kidneys, and cause kidney failure.

I go grab Emma in the lounge area. We walk quickly into Graham's room. Graham is shouting and mumbling at the top of his voice. Graham is blind in both eyes. He had one false left eye, and the other eye had gradually deteriorated since being on the unit. The nurses suspected he had a stroke and that had affected his eyesight further. Graham was of medium build, with a few tufts of grey hair. He was wearing a t-shirt that said 'Lucky Man', with an Irish clover leaf below. I couldn't decipher anything that Graham was shouting out. Gerry was standing over him looking more and more worried.

Gerry spoke to Emma and me.

'He's been doing this since I got here at teatime, just shaking and mumbling out loud, and his stomach is rock hard.'

Touching a resident's stomach area or abdomen can often be a good indicator of retention, particularly if it is hard to the touch.

We quickly move over to Graham and gradually take his tee shirt and vest off. They are soaked through with sweat and are damp to the touch, and hot. Graham continues to shout out incoherently.

'You ouououou, mmmmm yououououuoouou.'

'It's okay Dad' Gerry whispers nervously.

Once we had got Graham's shirt and vest off, we get him into the top half of his pyjamas. Emma walks off out of the room briefly to get the hoist. Graham was no longer able to walk, and had to be hoisted into his chair and bed. He had varying degrees of success in the stand aid, so the hoist was a much safer option.

Gerry continued to stay in the room with his dad. This made me a lot more nervous; you feel a lot more on show with relatives in the room. I have always felt a bit more nervy when such an occurrence presents itself. I had to remember I was a professional now, and had to act accordingly. Plus I really needed the toilet; somewhat ironic, given the current situation.

Emma comes briskly into the room with the hoist. She efficiently locks Graham into place, as we both clunk and click him into the hoist, effortlessly winching him up slowly, and moving him over to the bed. I walk around to the other side of the bed, and quickly help manoeuvre Graham into a safe central spot. We unclick the hoist, and gently roll him from one side to the next to undo the hoist.

Gerry is continually shouting out It's okay, his tone becoming more and more broken.

As I move Graham towards me, Emma quickly checks his pad.

'He's going to need changing.'

An acrid smell started to erupt into the room, slowly at first, and then more fierce. I tried to hold my breath without being too obvious, but it was too difficult to manage and concentrate on the task in hand, so I just kept on with short shallow breaths through my mouth. I could feel a stinging sensation against the back of my throat.

Emma rushes to the bathroom to get some wipes and towels. All the while I was clutching Graham with both hands, on his left hand side, and he was firmly pressed against my hips. He was starting to writhe around a little, and I offered him some words of assurance. Unfortunately the best I could come out with were not much better than his son's.

I could feel my arms beginning to ache. Graham's back was starting to become very hot and sweaty, and I could feel the heat rising up my own body as the situation continued. I was aware that Gerry was right on the other side of Graham, watching everyone's move. I didn't know where to look, so I continued to just say a few reassuring words to Graham and hope that Emma was quick in her accumulation of bathroom items.

She came back in a few mere seconds, clutching a bowl of hot soapy water and plenty of wipes. She started wiping around Grahams anus, cleaning him up, wipe by wipe. She had the professional air and the eye of a sculptor, working on her final masterpiece.

I balanced my furtive glances at either Graham, Emma, or Graham's son. I decided to give them ten seconds or so each, and try to keep as professional looking as possible. I wished a hole would open up in the ground soon, so that it could quickly swallow me and take me away from this very hot and seemingly crowded room. Suddenly my saviour was at the door, with two sharp knocks.

Paul quickly entered into the room clutching a variety of bright green boxes.

'Right, I think that's all we need, I've grabbed one of the nurses over the way who can catheterise, she should be along in a moment, how is he?'

'Still the same' Gerry answers. 'He's getting a lot more distressed, and shouting out.'

'Right, she won't be long, then we will get it sorted.'

Not everyone in the home could catheterise. As we saw this morning, if it was within certain hours, then an out of hours service would have to be called, however if there were general nurses on the other units who could catheterise then they would often be called upon to come and help out in situations like this. You would often feel a little powerless as a mental health nurse in these situations.

When at university, our mental health group would often get the odd jibe or ribbing as to what we 'actually did'. I remember clearly one day when I was sat in the lounge area at the university, one of the general nurses sidled up to me and came out with the question 'What is it you actually do then? Do you just play games all day long?'

What does a nurse do?

During my time at university, whilst on placement, I too was a little blinkered, viewing the nurses sat in the office, seemingly writing endless notes and reports. It was hard for me to clarify exactly what they did. Working in the nursing home, and being in charge of a unit, you started to realise exactly how much went on behind the scenes, and it wouldn't always be easy for others to see exactly what you had done in a day. The fact that it had been a smooth running shift would often be a good indicator. Often the carers would not witness the endless phone calls from relatives and to doctors. They wouldn't see the care plans you had written, the nursing notes that you had documented. Often carers would joke about how it was easy for a nurse, just 'sitting in the office' all the time or just 'doing the medication'.

They would appear to view themselves as having the real hard work. Caring was certainly no easy task, it was just as mentally and physically draining as being in charge of a shift. As the adage went, the nurses could do the carers' job, but the carers could not do the nurses' job. One day Sharon found this out.

When Sharon was working on one of the other units, she had taken rather a few liberties regarding her smoking breaks, and was trying to assert her authority to all the carers without consulting the nurse in charge. She had made the odd sly dig at the nurse (who had years of experience) about how she was always in the office. The nurse had finally had enough one day, and had decided that the next day Sharon would have the keys for the day.

The nurse did the morning medication the next day, then promptly handed Sharon the keys, and stated that

> Sharon could make all the decisions and answer all the phone calls. The nurse would be on hand to administer any dressings or medication, but it was down to Sharon for everything else. Sharon was completely shocked, but she took it in her stride and tried to do the best she could. She lasted two hours, and finally had to take the nurse to one side and apologise to her. She said she didn't appreciate the level of responsibility she had as a nurse, and would rather give the keys back; she had learnt her lesson.
>
> Sharon told everyone in the smoking shelter that the nurse had requested the keys back, but she hadn't. The nurse was quite prepared for Sharon to run the shift for the entire day. Sharon just wanted to save face in the smoking community. The nurse had highlighted just exactly how hard it can be working as a nurse. I would often joke about handing the keys to a carer, but not one of them would take me up on it. I think deep down they do realise how hard a job it can be, and if they are honest, not one of them wants to do it. I would often chat to the carers about whether they wanted to do their nurse training, and they would say the main reason for not doing it is that nurses never seemed to spend enough time with residents, and we always seemed to be locked away in the office. And they couldn't bear the thought of writing essays.

If everyone is thinking that way then mental health has a long way to go to change people's attitudes and perceptions about what is intrinsically valuable about your skills and role as a nurse.

A general nurse so eloquently phrased the question to me (after much smugness in telling me all about how she could re-catheterise and set up peg feeds);

'So what do you know then? What would be something you could tell me about mental health?'

'Well, you know if someone is hearing voices?

'Okay?'

'Do you want to know how to tell if they're just faking it, or if they are actually genuinely fearful and paranoid of their voices, and quite possibly psychotic?

'Sure.'

'Ask them if they have ever told their voices to piss off.'

'Why on earth would you say that?!'

'Well someone who is genuinely suffering from a form of psychosis and is hearing voices will do anything to get rid of their voices. They will swear at them, tell them to piss off, do anything they can to try and rid their voices from inside their head. Someone who is faking won't necessarily tell you that, they will often just say no. And that little fact is not something you will read about in the text books.'

'Thanks, I'll remember that!'

Just a little pearl of wisdom I had picked up from a placement area, and all of a sudden, from that moment on, I had started to gain a little more respect from the adult nurses.

Paul was looking a little anxious as we were all stood around Graham, as he was continuing to shout out and mumble to himself. Another knock at the door, and a incredibly tall, slim lady walked in, with short black hair. She was a general nurse from across the way. She had an air of authority about her as she stared through her dark rimmed spectacles.

Without hesitation, she started grabbing various boxes from Paul, and unpacked them. She then started to get to work. Much like what I had seen before with Edward, and just as excruciating, she took out the existing catheter pipe and reinserted a new one, after expertly pushing some anaesthetic gel straight up Graham's penis. Graham winced a little and continued to mumble throughout the whole procedure. I was holding Graham's hand, and he was gripping very tightly throughout. His son was looking over us all, wincing himself at every movement of the catheter pipe going in.

Once the new catheter was in, everyone stopped and stared at the leg bag, which up till now had drained barely a few millimetres of urine. A few seconds passed.

Nothing was happening. I could feel the tension in the room bearing down on us all like a lead weight.

There was a slight trickling sound, then all of a sudden a huge gush of urine started to fill the leg bag. The bag was suddenly bulging with urine; it had drained almost a litre of fluid, almost immediately. Graham seemed to let out a huge sigh of relief. He was not mumbling as much as before, the mumbles had dulled to a barely audible murmur. Everyone looked relieved.

The general nurse quickly walked out of the room. Paul looked relieved, and spoke to Gerry.

'He should be all right now, he'll probably just go to sleep, he seems a lot better after that, we drained almost a litre already.'

Gerry nodded. He looked more settled now, pleased that his dad was now not showing any signs of distress.

Paul, Emma, and I all nod to Gerry, and leave the room, leaving Graham to sleep off his recent ordeal.

Paul turns to Emma and me.

'All in days work eh? All in a day's work.'

It was now time to start putting people to bed. The carers would leap up for one last physical burst of energy. Most residents would be put to bed, with only a handful staying up for when the night staff came on. The hospital would work very differently to this, waiting for the night staff that came on to put everyone to bed, so that everyone went to bed around 10 p.m.

The partners who had paired up in the morning would work together again in the evening, if everything went to plan. This meant I was working with Emma again, and our first mission was to get Vancy into bed.

Vancy was sitting in the chair in the quiet lounge, fast asleep. Emma and I walk into the quiet lounge. Emma has a wheelchair ready. She gently stirs Vancy.

'Vancy, are you ready to go to bed?'

Vancy gradually opens her eyes, and looks at Emma.

'What love?'

'Would you like to go to bed Vancy?'

'Oh yes please love, that would be nice.'

Emma and I gradually help get Vancy to her feet, and then sit her in the wheelchair, and begin wheeling her to her bedroom.

As we are halfway down the corridor, Sharon comes walking up and shouts out down to us.

'We need a hand with Jim! He is biting and punching, and he has shredded his pad...We need a man.'

Sharon laughs to herself.

'Sure,' I say.

I walk up quickly with Sharon. As I enter Jim's room, I can see him awkwardly being stood up by Katie. Bits of his bright blue pad are strewn all across the floor. Jim's eyes are bulging, and he is drooling profusely. Sharon quickly attends to Jim's left side, so she and Katie are holding him upright.

'I've got the new pad ready, I just need you to take what's left of his old one off, and pop his new one on, and be very careful!'

I quickly spot the new pad on the bed, and walk up around to the front of Jim. He immediately starts to try and kick out at me. I move quickly and tear the tabs off the blue tag pad. It quickly falls to the floor and I grab the new pad, and quickly attach it to Jim.

Jim is starting to resist Katie and Sharon holding him. I can see both his arms bulging with veins.

'You can bloody stop now!'

'Almost done Jim, don't worry.'

The pad gets tagged into place, and I remove myself from Jim's front side. His legs are starting to kick out. Sharon and Katie effectively move him around quickly and sit him on the bed. Sharon whips Jim's legs up onto the bed, and raises the cot sides up on the bed and they snap into place. Jim tries to bite Sharon, but Sharon is too quick for him. She gently places a sheet over Jim, but Jim immediately starts grabbing hold of it and starts throwing it back onto the floor.

'Just leave him now, he will be like that for a while, at least he is safe, thank you love.'

I walk out of Jim's room. The last vision I see of Jim is him with his legs up in the air, and both hands in mid air, trying to hit out at the space in front of him, his eyes still bulging, his white wispy hair bedraggled.

I join Emma in Vancy's room. Vancy is a lot more settled than this morning, and is very compliant with Emma taking her clothes off and putting her night clothes on. Emma looks very stressed and tired.

'You alright?'

'Yeah, just tired. It's this job, I know you're new and everything, but I've got to get out of here, no one supports you, and it's just getting worse.'

'What's the worst thing about the place?'

'Oh you don't want to know, you don't want to hear my troubles about this place.'

'I'd rather you be honest with me, it's good to know what's happening.'

'Well, it's just morale, there's no team work any more, people just do what they like, and things are getting missed, and it's the residents who are losing out in the end. I've been in this job too long, and I'm getting out, it's becoming a chore, coming to work each day, and that's a sign I need to move on.'

'Right.'

'Take this whole teamwork crap. It's a joke, people like Sharon and Katie just do their own thing anyway, they will put residents to bed who are the 'easier' people, and they will always grab the laundry trolley after they have put people to bed, so they can go down for a quick last cigarette, even though it is frowned upon by the management. No one should need a cigarette at 7:30, when they finish work at 8.'

'And does this happen every evening?'

'Pretty much. Not once do I take the laundry trolley down, I don't even have a chance, they rule this place, and no one cares. The other day two baths got missed, and the carers just covered it up, pretending they didn't have the time. One of those baths was highly important as was a part of a resident's treatment, as he has really bad psoriasis of the legs. When I confronted those involved they denied it. They said that they had bathed the residents. It's disgusting, it is. You better watch that Sharon too, she will order you around and tell you who she wants put into bed, but stand up to her, and don't work on your own if you don't want to; I wouldn't.'

I was shocked yet pleased I was getting the run-down of the unit, and what was really going on.

'Let's just watch them tonight. They will often not use the proper equipment. Frequently they will put people into bed without using either the stand aid or the hoist, because it is quicker, easier, and less time consuming. Everything is becoming one big race here.

It is supposed to be twenty four hour care. But that's a joke. I've seen people wheel residents around in stand aids up the corridor. It's so undignified; everything done to cut corners.'

'What can be done about it?'

'That's the trouble, seemingly nothing, people like Sharon have all the power, they bulldoze you into thinking their way, and they get away with it.'

Emma paused.

'But something's going to change, it's got to, I'm not putting up with it any more, I refuse to let people boss me about and treat me like fucking dirt. This ends tonight.'

7–8 p.m.

Paul was in the corridor speaking to Gerry.

'How long you been married then Paul?'

'Oh going on for about fifteen years now, very happily married, how about yourself?'

'Not for me, never fancied it myself, it's just a bit of paper at the end of the day, but fair play to you for getting on with it. I just never got round to it!'

They both laughed out loud. A bit of harmless banter was always a good way to build rapport with the relatives. What might be seen as simply having a chat, would further reinforce the work of relationship centred care.

Relationship centred care

'Relationship centred care is healthcare that values and attends to the relationships that form the context of care **(Caring Matters, 2005)**. Relationship centred concepts were born out of person centred approaches, but helps develop this more by working in partnership with family and carers and developing this relationship alongside the patient.

'The notion of relationship extends beyond just three people to other members of the care team, which can include not only family members but also professionals' **(Adams, 2005)**. 'Alongside medical treatment, effort should be put into establishing a relationship with the individual that ensures their needs will be heard and responded too.' **(Parliamentary and Health Service Ombudsman, 2011).**

As Paul and Gerry were finishing their conversation on marriage, Ian started walking up the corridor. He walks straight past them, but not before giving them both a quick glance.

'I'm innocent!'

Ian carries on walking up the corridor. Both Paul and Gerry turn around to Ian, and laugh out loud. Whether Ian had actually heard the conversation or not was hard to tell, but there were genuine moments within mental health whereby residents could really come out with some quite accurate and insightful comments. These were the moments to cherish, above the anguish and sometimes desperate air that could lie thick within the unit. How many times had we heard the old adage 'If you don't laugh, you would cry'? How many times would that ring in my ears, as my career progressed and developed, and invited me to new and challenging experiences.

Ian continues to walk all the way up the corridor, tries the exit door a few times, and quickly turns around and starts walking up towards me.

'Hey sir!'

Ian was walking a little unsteadily up the corridor. He had his stick in his hand, but still looked surprisingly unsteady.

'Hi Ian, how can I help?'

'I'm trying to find the way out, and the toilet'

'The toilet is this way Ian.'

I point, and Ian slowly walks into the toilet.

'Will you wait for me then? I want a word with you afterwards, I want you to run me up the road.'

'Sure, I will wait here for you, don't worry.'

I wait a few moments outside the toilet. I start to read the notice board in front of me. There are a few cards from relatives thanking the unit for all their hard work looking after their father or mother during their last hours. A few clicks and a flush later, Ian is standing outside the toilet with me. His eyes look eager.

'Right, show me the way then.'

'Where?'

'To go home!'

'Ian, I have to work here till eight I am afraid, why don't we sit in the office a while?'

'Well all right then.'

Ian dutifully follows me into the nursing office and sits down. Paul is just finishing off the evening medication. I can hear him whistling away to himself further up the corridor.

'Right Ian, what shall we do, would you like a drink?'

'Well I wouldn't mind, what are you offering?'

'Tea, coffee?'

'Have you got anything stronger?'

There was a selection of alcoholic drinks locked away in the medicine cupboard in the office, most of which had been donated by relatives over numerous Christmases. The doctors had agreed that everyone was entitled to a little tipple now and again. Christmas was traditionally a time for giving. Most of the relatives would present the unit with bottles of wine and boxes of biscuits, to be distributed amongst the staff who had been looking after their relatives over the past year. One relative specifically bought a bottle of wine for each member of staff on the unit.

One year, management decided that this was not fair on the other units, and confiscated the bottles of wine and distributed them over the whole home, to all staff members, including office staff (who traditionally get most of the Christmas week off, and have no direct contact with any residents). The relatives found out about this and were furious. Gifts were being given to staff members that they had never met or intended to give to. There had also been some small monetary donations given to units, with the express purpose of giving the unit staff a night out, but again, the management confiscated this money, and stated that it could be considered a bribe from the relatives. The money was kept by management.

'Well, there is whisky, wine and sherry in the cupboard actually, are you a whisky man?'

'Yep, whisky will be fine my good man, don't be shy about the amount either, I'll have one of those then please.'

'Okay.'

I quickly walk out of the office and grab the keys off Paul. I unlock the cupboard, and pour a small shot of whisky out for Ian.

'Would you like anything else with it?'

'Yeah, fill it with a bit of water will you?'

I fill the whisky up with water and hand it back to Ian.

'There you go, enjoy.'

'Thank you kind sir.'

Ian gulps back the whisky and water, and smiles.

'That hits the spot all right, have you got any more?'

'I might be able to get you some more. Let's relax a minute for now, have you had a good day today, have you settled in okay?'

Ian looks a little confused for a while.

'Well, it's been all right I guess, but things aren't the same as they used to be.'

'I know Ian, it's hard, but we are all here to look after you.'

'It's a lovely building this though isn't it, they must have done a good job here, very nice indeed, how long have you worked here?'

'It's my first day today.'

'Is it really? I thought you had worked here longer than that!'

'No.'

'Well, I think you will get used to it, they seem nice people around here, and it's good service.'

'It certainly seems so.'

'Have you seen Roger today?'

'No, who is Roger?'

'You know Roger, he's one of your mates too, I wanted to catch up with him today, we were going to do some work together, and if I don't find him I won't know what we have left to do.'

'I think he has gone home actually.'

'Oh, that's a shame, I could have done with catching up, oh well, I will get him tomorrow I expect.'

'How long were you in the plastering trade Ian?'

'What do you mean, how long?'

'How long did you work for?'

'I don't understand you.'

'How long were you a plasterer?'

'I still am!'

'Oh, right, how long have you been doing it so far then?'

'Well, I wouldn't like to say, years and years, can I have another whisky?'

'Another whisky! You had that one a bit quick Ian, you will get me into trouble!'

'Well, I won't say anything if you won't, go on, give me a good measure, and I will see you right.'

'You like your whisky then!'

'Oh yes, I'm a bit partial to a drop of wine now and again, but whisky is my favourite.'

I appreciated Ian's brutal honesty, and poured him a very small measure of whisky, and again filled it right up with water, and placed the cup back into his hand.

'Thanks fella, I'll see you right don't you worry, I see all my best friends right.'

Ian quickly drinks the whisky, and stands up.

'Right, I'm off, I'm going to have a bit of a walk.'

He extends his right arm out to me, and I shake it.

'Thanks fella, I'll see you tomorrow, what time are you coming in?'

'I will be here at 8 a.m. sharp.'

'8 a.m. sharp?! Right, well I'm going to make it for about 8:30 then okay?'

'Yep, that's fine, we will have a coffee together, does that sound good?'

'Brilliant, sounds good to me! See you tomorrow then!'

I can still hear the faint whistles of Paul up the corridor. I go to return the keys to him. Katie and Sharon are bustling away, still putting people to bed.

Paul had finished up the medication and was wheeling the medication trolley back down towards me. He locks it away in a small cubby hole. He glances at a large frame full of pictures of residents and staff members.

'I think they had better change some of these pictures you know, half of them are dead! Doesn't look good for the other relatives really.'

He looks the pictures up and down once more, and spots a picture of Sally, grinning with another resident.

'There she is, the Citalopram kid, yee hah!'

Paul shapes his fingers into small pistols, and re-enacts an imaginary wild west shoot out, and walks into the nursing office. As soon as he sits down the phone rings.

He turns to me.

'I'll bet you a thousand pounds it's Sindy asking about Jim.'

Before I could answer him, he picked up the phone.

'Hello, Franklyn unit, Paul speaking'

Paul smiles and turns towards me as the phone is still wedged tightly against his ear.

'Sindy, how are you! Yes he has had a good day, he's been in his room today, a little agitated at times when taking his medication, but overall no real changes with him, but he has eaten and drunk well.'

Paul continues with the phone conversation.

'Yes, I will no problem, and thank you, speak to you tomorrow.'

Paul puts the phone down.

'Sindy's nice. Rings on the dot, every evening without fail. You get to know your relatives and how to handle them. Mark my words though, no matter how good a relationship you build with them, if they have any doubts with the care of their relatives, they will soon turn on you. I have seen it happen, so treat them fairly, but always be aware that at the back of your mind, they can be your own worst enemy. Just document everything, and communicate with them. There's nothing more you can do really, just cover yourself, that's what the job's getting like these days. Always cover your back, and document everything, and you have nothing to worry about.'

The phone immediately goes again. Paul sighs, and picks it up. After a few mumbles and 'uhums', Paul slams the phone back down, lets out a large sigh and turns to me.

'There's no staff for tomorrow, they're only going to be running on four staff all day, three carers and one nurse, and I think we need at least one extra for the unit.'

'Oh, that's no good,' I say.

'I've tried everyone I can think of, I have rung everyone that usually cover extra shifts, and I have rung the unit manager at home, and because it's a weekend Jennifer won't authorise me to pay for agency staff.'

I looked at Paul a bit puzzled.

'She won't what?'

'She told me specifically that she couldn't authorise to pay for agency staff because it was on a weekend.'

'Is this a new thing they have started then?'

'No idea, but that's what Jennifer has told me, and has overall say on the matter, so they're going to run short tomorrow, and with an unknown quantity in our new resident, technically we can run on four staff, even though this is the heaviest unit and we need at least five.'

'I'd better ring the nurse in charge tomorrow. He's on his own; best break the bad news to him gently.'

'That's shocking that they won't do that,' I say.

'Yep, seems about right for this place you know, the trouble is Ian is a totally unknown quantity, he's quite settled at present, but I have heard he can be quite aggressive and quite capable of running down the corridor and being physically aggressive towards people at a moment's notice.'

'So under no circumstances will they pay for agency staff?'

'Not at all mate, nothing more I can do I'm afraid.'

'What does that mean then?'

'Well, it just means the nurse will be absolutely pushed all day long. The carers will feel the pinch as it means that one carer will have to work on her own getting people up, which you shouldn't be having to, and the nurse will have to try and help out as much as he can, but it's hard going at the best of times, and really we shouldn't be put in this situation at all. It just goes to show you kid, that it's all about money when it comes down to it.'

'Wow, that is incredible.'

'Ain't it just...Ain't it just? You should look at getting into the NHS you know. They have their problems I know, but you won't really learn anything here, you will be constantly trying to put out fires, and they will take the piss out of you. You're just a number to them, they would replace you tomorrow, but don't let me put you off again! I have a habit of doing that!'

Ian comes walking back into the nursing station. At this time of the evening it would be common for people to be a bit more alert and start wandering.

'Hey what's going on in here then? You two fellas are always about!'

'We sure are,' smiles Paul.

'Keep taking the pills I say, that's all we can do, and keep going.'

There is a random roll of toilet paper in the office. The office would often be used as a dumping ground for random bits of paper, hair curlers, combs, watches, glasses. You name it, everything got left in the office, and usually stayed there for a number of months.

Paul grabs the toilet paper and shows it to Ian.

'Hey Ian, can I give you this, just in case you get caught short?'

Ian looks and smiles at me, then at Paul.

'You're a bugger you are!'

Ian turns back to me.

'Do you have to put up with him every day like this?' I smile.

'Yeah, I think I will have to.'

'I don't know how you do it, he's a bugger alright.'

Paul smiles back at Ian.

'Hey Ian, you're just like me aren't you, we both have a few miles on the clock.'

'Yep, I've been around a bit, I could tell you a few things.'

Ian gives Paul a look up and down.

'Mind you, you look as though you're getting on a bit.'

Paul laughs out loud.

'I am, and you'll be giving me more grey hairs!'

Ian smiles.

'Get out! You have quite a few already you know!'

'Oh I know,' Paul laughs.

'You look like you eat well,' Ian smiles at Paul.

Paul quickly walks out of the nursing station, and goes to grab an apple from the fruit bowl in the kitchen, and returns with it.

'Hey Ian, fancy an apple?'

'Well, I wouldn't say no!'

Ian takes hold of the apple, and starts biting into it, at a terrific pace. A few moments pass. Paul tries to tidy up the nursing station a little, putting the books in order on the shelf above him. Ian is still eating the apple, and starting to eat the core, with the pips still intact. In fact, devouring the entire apple. I look at Ian in disbelief.

'Ian, are you enjoying that apple?'

'Yep.'

Ian seems oblivious to the fact that he is eating the hard apple core and pips, and continues on till there is nothing left of the apple.

Paul turns back to Ian, and puts his fists up in a jokey manner.

'Put 'em up Ian.'

Ian looks at Paul and smiles.

'Hark at him, I could knock you down with one fell swoop mister! I'd give you a good smack in the chops!'

'You don't really want to hit me do you Ian? What about all those jobs we have to do tomorrow?'

'Yes, that's true, well when are we going to sort them then?'

'In the morning. How much do you think we could charge?'

Ian smiles.

'Well I don't know, but we need a fair price that's for sure, but the job will be quality that's for sure.'

'Of course, I agree.'

Ian laughs out loud.

Paul had tapped into his humour, and it was working. He was a true inspiration.

Ian was smiling at the both of us. His smile seemed completely genuine, and for a brief second you could forget all about his illness, and the sometimes cruel and dark nature of it; he was Ian, Ian the plasterer, he had a life, and he had a history, and we were learning more and more about him as the hours went on. It was at times like this I would think how great it would be to just take people like Ian down to the local pub, and have a good chat with him, give him something to really savour and enjoy, and for one brief moment, take him out of this sometimes mundane existence, and evoke a sense of hope.

This is what mental health was supposed to be about. I had learnt it from my lecturers. It didn't always go the way you would like, but I knew that inspiration and hope were the key areas, for the people that were in your care. It was so sad at times that you couldn't really do the things you wanted to do as a mental health nurse, always having constraints and procedure to follow first, that would detract from your time with any of your residents. University showed you the perfect model of care.

I lost count of the mentors I had worked with who had ground me down, week after week, telling me that it wasn't like it was at university, and that I had to live in the real world, amongst paperwork, and potential litigation every day of the week. It shouldn't have to be that way, there shouldn't be this huge practice gap between education and the work environment. But only we could change it, one small step at a time. As Lao Tzu once said:

'Prepare for the difficult while it is still easy; deal with the big while it is still small.'

Ian would come to be a big part of the unit, and eventually give Paul another dilemma in the use of Benperidol. Over the months, Ian would start to grab hold of some of the other female residents on the unit, initially grabbing of hands, trying to redirect them to other areas of the unit. Other times he would grab a little harder, and startle other female residents, but it was all done without any malice intended. One of the female residents would remind Ian a little of his wife, and he would think he was sharing moments with his wife.

One of the relatives took umbrage with the amount of time Ian seemed to be spending around his wife, and complained to the nurse in charge. As a result, the next ward round Ian was put on Benperidol.

The drug regime continued for a number of weeks. But Ian still remained a little playful at times and still maintained some hand touching and grabbing with the same female residents, but it wasn't just localised to females, he would often take the hand of male residents on the unit.

On the next ward round, the Benperidol was doubled. Ian continued in his behaviour. Ian had a girlfriend who visited the unit regularly. She had also requested the use of the room key, and the ability to lock the room, with both her and Ian inside it.

This highlighted particular implications. Did Ian have the capacity for sexual preferences, was he able to understand the difference, able to make a well informed choice? There was no proof that anything was going on with them in his room, but we as nurses have a duty of care to help promote an individual's sexuality and preferences as long as they maintain the capacity to make informed choices and decisions. Ian, it was deemed, had the capacity to make these choices, and so the key was given to the girlfriend when she visited. As two consenting adults they would be entitled to do what they liked in the privacy of Ian's room as long as this capacity remained.

Meanwhile Ian was still on the Benperidol, a drug that was trying to curb his sexual inappropriateness, whilst we were promoting his own sexuality, allowing him to have private time with his girlfriend. The girlfriend was made aware of the medication changes, as she remained an important part of Ian's life, and all of Ian's daughters agreed that the girlfriend could be informed of any changes. The situation would carry on, continuing with a medication that curbed sexual inappropriateness, whilst simultaneously having visits from a girlfriend. In an ideal world, having more staff on in the daytime would mean more one on one time with Ian, working towards distracting him and spending quality time together.

This was not the ideal world. Without enough staff members around, Ian would have the time to wander and invade the other residents' personal space. Without any facilities for non medical interventions, medical interventions would usually win out. Staff the unit to minimum recommendations, thus provide less opportunities for time with residents (i.e. taking Ian off the unit and into the garden area) so residents become more agitated and potentially aggressive, thus requiring medical input.

Paul turned to me.

'Don't spend too much time in your room or the Citalopram kid will have you, and don't touch anyone, or you will be put on Benperidol!' Paul laughed sarcastically.

These were serious medications being given to people. These were people's lives we were dealing with, and drugs had considerable side effects.

I could hear a lot of clanking and commotion from outside the corridor, and Sharon's loud booming voice. She was shouting to Emma.

'Emma, how are you doing that end love ? Listen, I would take Elsie to bed next okay baby, she will only moan and complain if not.'

There was a slight pause. I could almost see tension building, like a very thick mist wrapping itself around Emma and Sharon.

'No Sharon, I'm not doing it.'

'Your what?'

'No, I'm sorry, I'm not working on my own tonight doing Elsie. I do it every night, and I'm not putting up with it. It's not fair on the residents, I will wait till someone can give me a hand, I can't be doing with it.'

A very long pause ensued.

'Ohhhhh, okay then, I'm sorry I asked, well we are going to Andrew next, so then the stand aid will be free if you need it.'

I could hear Sharon wheeling the stand aid up the corridor. It rattled like an intercity train on the carpet. There would often be a slight sense of stress in the air, whilst people were being put to bed.

No matter how many times management had told the carers that it was 'twenty four hour care', the slight panic always seemed to ensue about how many residents needed to be safely put into bed, so there would often be quite a commotion and clanking of moving and handling equipment, as people were popped into bed, like a bizarre production line.

Most would finish around 7:30 – 7:45 p.m. Sometimes some staff would often tweak the times that they started getting residents into bed, and start as early as 6:10 p.m., whereas most staff would start sensibly, no earlier than 6:30 p.m.

On most evenings, the staff would be finished just in time to catch the last of Eastenders or Emmerdale and have one last cup of tea or coffee. This was the final way to wind down after a long shift.

Everyone was stretched beyond their capabilities. There would be the occasional meeting held, when it got to breaking point, and the manager of the unit would call it. Everyone would be paid for their time at the meeting, but a lot of the staff wouldn't turn up, despite them having a lot to say during their shifts on the unit, and how they wished things would change. A typical meeting would last around an hour. Usually nothing would really change, but it provided a good sounding board for people to vent their opinions.

Typical topics for a meeting:

Pillows - There were never enough pillows on the unit. We used a lot of pillows, due to many being used to help turn and reposition residents in bed, to keep them off their pressure sore areas.

Eating off the trolley - The main argument from the carers was that the actual person in charge of the kitchen didn't care if the carers ate off the trolley. The eggs and bacon were literally going to get thrown away in the bin. The management had reached a semi agreement. There was now no problem with anyone eating a 'singular' egg or round of bacon. The issue was with making sandwiches, and using up the bread from the unit. If all the carers made themselves egg sandwiches every morning, then this could constitute a couple of loaves every day, and this was not acceptable. Having an egg would now be fine, as long as it was on its own.

People were still being seen to be making sandwiches, the last example being of the young upstart sat eating a bacon sandwich at around nine in the morning, right in the middle of the lounge area. Unfortunately for her, this was the exact time that the manager of the home walked through, and caught her eating it. She never said anything to the upstart, but merely went straight to Paul, and gave him a roasting about why people were eating off the trolley still; there was, she said, absolutely no call for it.

Unbeknownst to the manager, Paul accepted the roasting, with the small greasy remains of a bacon sandwich in his own front pocket. He had heard the crashing of the door to the unit, and quickly popped the sandwich into his pocket, quickly swallowing what he had in his mouth, before turning round to greet the manager. This was experience talking.

This was not the first time that Paul had to act quickly during his career. Many a sandwich or egg had to disappear quickly, like a magician's act. Paul once had to swallow an entire hot sausage straight down his gullet when an area manager had stepped onto his unit in the hospital where he was working. There wasn't much you could get past Paul. And the upstart would have a lot to learn about concealing food items, if you were going to continue to take things from the trolley. Experience certainly paved the way forward.

Chiropody appointments - Feet were a particular bugbear of the unit. Elderly residents would often have a lot of rough scaly skin, hard, irregular sized nails, and generally be in poor condition. Diabetics' feet were of particular importance. They are much more likely to develop foot ulcers. Diabetes can lead to poor circulation, and in particular a reduced feeling in the feet. There used to be a chiropodist who visited regular on the unit, but as time had pressed on, she had become a lot trickier to track down.

A list was maintained in the nursing station of everyone's feet that needed looking at. This list would develop over a few months, until there were at least ten residents on it. It would then be the job of the nurse to try and track down the chiropodist, who lived in the deepest darkest part of the country and could never be found, despite numerous phone calls and messages. She would charge ten pounds per foot. Recently it had come to light that it wasn't actually the nurses' or the home's responsibility to provide this service. From now on everyone had to explain to the relatives that it needed to be their responsibility to find their own chiropodist, just like they would have to do with dentists.

Lounge left unattended for long periods when staff are in bedrooms – this is felt to be dangerous - When carers were helping people in their rooms, either in the morning getting them up, or attending to the residents who needed changing and repositioning in their bed in the afternoon, this could mean that the lounge area was left unattended for long periods of time. A handful of residents would always be in the lounge area, and some of them could start to wander, and some were very liable to fall.

If anything happened, there wouldn't be anyone in the lounge area to help. Risk can never be eliminated, merely minimised. One way around this was to make sure the nurse was in the lounge area doing their nursing notes from about 3 p.m. onwards. The notes would take at least an hour, and this would at least provide another person in the lounge area, who could help keep an eye on things. Of course this wouldn't always be possible if the nurse had to deal with other issues.

Dirty carpets and stained chairs - the chairs and carpets were totally filthy in most of the rooms. Having spoken to the many cleaners on the unit, this came down to the fact that the home only supplied standard household cleaning appliances and chemicals. To clean the carpets and chairs of a well used nursing home required something with a little more kick to it, an industrial based solution. This was not something that the home was currently prepared to pay for. All the units had been promised a roll out of new plastic based furniture, which would be far easier to clean and maintain.

More spoons and small bowls - There were much more residents requiring being fed, as their dementia deteriorated and required much more one to one assistance. This meant more bowls and spoons were needed in order to assist the residents with their most basic need.

Restocking bedrooms at night - The incontinence pads were now starting to be stocked during the night shifts, so they would be ready for the whole day's shift. This didn't always seem to work, as during the day they would frequently run out of pads towards the evening. Due to the variable nature of general continence amongst residents, the amount of pads would often vary on a daily basis.

Teamwork – e.g. – Ensuring both sides have completed all jobs together – A continual struggle, and one that would probably never be solved. No matter how many times this was explained to the staff, they would still find a way to get out of working together. The official standing still stood that getting residents up in the morning should be a team effort. Once a side was completed, then it was up to the other team to go and help whoever else needed to be got up.

Laundry trolley in the evening - The carers were still at it. When they had finished putting people to bed of an evening, the smokers would be the first ones to declare that they were taking the laundry trolley down of an evening. Their job was to simply empty the yellow clinical waste bags into the large yellow clinical waste bins, and to leave the full laundry bags in the laundry, next to the washing machines. This was starting to take far too long of an evening, mainly due to the carers having one last crafty cigarette, before coming back up onto the unit. The excuses carried on as to why they were so long of an evening for such a menial task.

Some of the carers liked to physically load the washing machines up ready for the next morning, even though it was not in their job description. Others used to sweep the smoking shelter area clear of any stray cigarette ends, despite there being clearly marked bins for this purpose. All these appeared to be excuses to waste a little more time in order for the carers to have one last drag of a cigarette before returning back onto the unit. One last hit of nicotine, before they finished work, despite the fact that their shift was due to end in approximately twenty minutes.

Jennifer would eventually have enough of people smoking, and really put her foot down. A male carer, Jason, was caught one last time, having a sly cigarette whilst taking the laundry down. She sacked him on the spot. His attitude was appalling. Ironically he was leaving in two weeks; he was off to an acute service, to work with younger adults. As soon as he was fired, he stormed off the unit and punched the wall hard enough to make a small indentation. This sent ripples through the smoking community, and put them on edge, and really tightened up the control of the smokers and how many liberties they were really willing to take. It was the final straw. An email then went around the home and further sent the message home:

'Staff have to understand that breaks are at the allotted time each day as indicated on the daily work sheet. There must be no smoking breaks after breakfast.'

They had begun to monitor people's whereabouts by CCTV. They ruled that if any staff were seen to be smoking outside any allotted breaks then it would result in disciplinary action and probable dismissal.

It was up to nurses to keep everyone in check and notify Jennifer if any further staff were still going out and catching a quick smoking break. This was unfair on the carers that did not smoke.

Any other business - One last chance to try to suggest ways to change things, but ultimately things wouldn't change. You either hated it but got on with it, or you left to get another job. The management would love to remind the staff that around five to six people rang the home each and every day to enquire about whether there were any jobs going. The bottom line being, everyone should be lucky that they had a job, and if they didn't like it, they knew where the exit doors were.

I walk out onto the corridor, and place a handful of dirty socks and pants into the patient clothing laundry bag. Emma comes quickly behind me.

'Come on, let's quickly get Bob into bed, then we can take the laundry trolley down, and beat Sharon and Katie to it for once!'

'Okay.'

We quickly march up the corridor, and into Bob's room. Bob is fast asleep in his chair, with both hands outstretched, and up in the air, like he is climbing an imaginary ladder.

'Bob, we just need to put you into bed, you don't look very comfortable like that.'

Bob continues to have his eyes shut.

We carefully help Bob up onto his feet. I ease off his slippers and socks, Emma pops his head down comfortably onto the pillow, and we click the cot sides up into place.

As we are doing this we can hear the faint rattle of the laundry trolley coming up the corridor. Emma glances at me. I look at her, then into the corridor.

The trolley sound is getting louder. Sharon shouts out from behind the door.

'We're just taking the trolley down now okay baby?'

I could see the look of sadness erupt over Emma's face. The sound of the trolley gradually fades as Sharon and Katie guide it up the corridor, and out off the unit.

Emma turns to me.

'Fucking hell, those two must have hearing like bats.'

We walk out of Bob's room, after putting on his portable CD player. Most of the residents had their own music players in their room, and it often seemed to settle them to sleep. Often the staff would put the music on for them in the morning too.

'Goodnight Bob.'

Bob doesn't really stir.

I try next.

'Goodnight Bob.'

We walk out of the room, leaving the door open. I look at my watch: 7:37 p.m. There would be no more time to put anyone else to bed. Everyone was in bed, who normally would go to bed. Emma offers me a final drink of the day.

'I'll have a coffee please.'

'No problems, milk no sugar isn't it?'

'Yes, thanks, what about Sharon and Katie?'

'Oh well, they can make their own. I'll ask Jenny, but those two are going down for a sneaky cigarette, so they can get theirs when they come back up. I don't see why we should wait on them.'

'Okay.'

Paul has finished the evening medication. He is sitting in the office, finalising the daily handover sheet, ready to discuss with the night nurse. I hover around the nursing station door; Jenny is sat in the quiet lounge, waiting patiently for debrief. Paul looks up at me.

'How has it gone today then mate? Are you enjoying it? You have certainly had a baptism of fire today, that's for sure.'

'Yeah, it has been an adventure.'

'Sure has, ready to do it all again tomorrow eh!'

'Yeah.'

Ian comes strolling past the office again and looks at Paul.

'Here he is, King Kong!'

He turns to me and smiles.

'And Acker Bilk!'

He laughs to himself.

'Hey can you tell me where the toilet is fellas?'

'Sure, just turn around, and it's the first door on your left Ian, just round the corner,' Paul says.

Ian turns around, and makes his way around the corner. Paul walks out of the office and towards the lounge area.

'Right, I've got an idea' Paul says. He quickly returns, clutching an acoustic guitar, crude in its appearance, and missing one string. Paul starts strumming away.

'Can you play?'

'Only a little, I know the main chords though, enough to get me by, it's all I really need.'

Right on cue, Ian walks around the corner again, and stops in the doorway as Paul is strumming away on the guitar. Ian seems perplexed yet fascinated by Paul's playing. A broad smile erupts over his face.

'Any request Ian?' Ian turns to me, as Paul continues to strum away, and starts singing Hey Jude.

'He's not too bad at all really is he?'

Paul is enthusiastically playing the guitar, singing a variety of well known songs, from the Rolling Stones to The Animals. Bob walks past the nursing office, and Ian shouts out to him as he passes.

'75p a ticket! This guy is really good!' Ian points at Paul and grins. Ian leans against the door of the nursing office, laughing at times, a low crackly laugh, becoming absorbed in Paul's guitar playing, watching intently as Paul continues to play through various well known classics. Ian points to Paul.

'Hey, listen fella, can I ask you something ?'

'Sure thing Ian.'

'Is it Okay if I stay here tonight?'

'Course you can, more than welcome.'

'Thank god for that, some cunts nicked my bike.'

Emma comes back down the corridor with a tray full of drinks. She puts a cup in the office for Paul.

'Here you are my lovely, tea no sugar.'

'You're an absolute star love, thanks. Now then, have we got time for a debrief? Where are Sharon and Katie, or need I ask?' Paul continues to play the guitar whilst speaking to Emma, enthusiastically strumming away. He eventually stops and leans the guitar against the office door.

'The usual?' Emma pipes up.

'Right, well there haven't been many changes anyway, depends when they get back really, how have things been today anyway Emma?'

'Same old...I'm still getting out of here, I've applied for a couple of jobs, it's got so bad here lately.'

'I know kid, morale has certainly hit the floor, I'll give you that.'

'I have just lost the passion Paul, and that's not fair on these residents. Everything else has ground me down, the politics, the staff, the management, everything has started to just grind, each and every single day.'

Ian straightens his glasses, and starts walking away from the nursing office.

'Can anyone tell me where the toilet is please?'

'Just round the corner Ian, first door on the left mate.'

'Okay, thanks.' Ian starts walking around the corner, past the nursing office window, and straight past the toilet door.

Jenny pops her head around the corner.

'How do Paul, are you tired?'

'I sure am Jenny. How's it going, any problems today?'

'There are always problems.'

She laughs, a dry laugh.

'How do you think Jack has got on today, have you shown him the ropes?'

'Yes, he can stay all right. Whether he wants to or not is another matter!' Emma smiles.

'You like a challenge though, eh Jack!'

'Oh yeah, I'll give it a go alright.'

Everyone laughs together.

A faint bang of the unit doors can be heard off in the distance. 7:48 p.m. I could hear Sharon talking to Katie halfway up the corridor. They bound enthusiastically down the corridor, and past the nursing station.

'Hello everyone, are we alright then?'

'Yes,' everyone answers in unison.

'Right, what's happening then?! Are we having a debrief or what? Oh I see, everyone got a cup of tea I see! It's like that is it?'

Sharon laughs, but you could tell deep down that she wasn't overly impressed, that no-one had made her a cup of tea.

Paul shuffles some paper in his hand.

'There's not a great deal to say ladies to be fair, we just have to keep our eyes on Daniel, and see if he is getting any more verbally aggressive, and if we notice any change. Jilly has had some eye drops ordered, as she keeps rubbing them and they are really red, and Mindy is having her Olanzapine increased, that's if you can get her to take it in the first place of course!'

Everyone nods at the brief knowledge gained about the residents.

Another click of the door, and some more steps can be heard. It is Hannah. She is here for another twelve hour night shift. She slowly puts her coat away in the store room, and walks up to everyone around the nursing station.

'All right Hannah, how is everything? How are you?' Paul asks.

'Not very well actually. I almost didn't come to work this evening in all honesty, I feel like shit.'

Everyone who was previously smiling now looks down and away from Hannah.

'Sorry to hear that Hannah, chin up love.'

'Yeah, I'll be all right, I've just a lot going on with my ex and my kids, anyway, I'm off to make a coffee.'

Hannah walks off to the kitchen area. Hannah would often have incredibly detailed chats with most of the nursing staff about her private life. She probably had enough material to write her own Mills and Boon romance, she had the makings of the next Barbara Cartland, if only she had the will to put it all down on paper.

Many a night staff carer would listen to her entire life story whilst sat in the lounge on a twelve hour shift. Fascinating at times, scary at others. Hannah was a good solid worker, and she knew her stuff, but she, like others, was looking for an exit strategy. She was in the middle of applying for jobs for other nursing homes a bit closer to home. She had also got wound down by the general policies and procedures, and how staff got treated here, and she wasn't afraid to tell anyone how she really felt, including the management. She was biding her time until she could get a new job and find her feet again.

Katie and Sharon had already gone to get their coats ready in preparation for the end of the shift. Carers were often incredibly precise at leaving on time, sometimes waiting downstairs by the reception area to clock off a few minutes before eight. This had been stopped of late, as one evening the owner of the home was standing at the reception area in readiness and gave everyone a good telling off. It didn't help that each clock in the home told a slightly different time, but the carers would often work out the one that gave them the most benefit.

The nurses would often stay till around 8:45-9 p.m., depending on how busy the shift had been. The minimal handover time would be about fifteen minutes, but it was often half an hour with ease to do it properly. The nurses would get paid for their extra time, but only fifteen minutes for one handover, and up to half an hour if the night nurse was running two floors. If you were late for any other reason you had to get it signed by Jennifer and explain your reasons why the handover took longer than the allotted fifteen minutes.

Sharon looked down at her watch.

'Right, I'm going down to wait by reception, okay baby,' she shouted at Paul. Paul wasn't interested. He let Sharon go, she was going to go anyway, whether he liked it or not. Katie followed like an obedient lap dog. Jenny and Emma were finishing their cups of tea.

Paul turns to me.

'Well matey, I guess I'll see you tomorrow then? That's if you want to come back of course?'

I pause a few seconds.

'Yeah, I'll be back...I get the feeling I'm going to have a challenge on my hands...But I will be back.'

I grab my bag and coat, and walk up the corridor with Jenny and Emma. I glance into the rooms, and see the residents flat out in their beds, each one completely at peace.

As I shut the unit door behind me I can see Ian walking up the corridor, fully clothed, and with his pyjamas over the top of his shirt, and his dressing gown. He is waving up the corridor shouting out.

'Wait for me! I want to go up the road!'

I walk to the exit door, and press the numbers on the key panel. The door shuts behind me and I look back through the small window of the door. Ian is there waving at me, trying the door handle, and banging on the door lightly. I can still hear him faintly through the door.

'Come on, let me out, run me up the road.'

'I'll be back soon Ian, I promise!'

Ian looks dejected, and continues to bang on the door.

I walk down the stairs. I can still faintly hear his banging on the door. I clock out by reception. Most of the carers are long gone by now. I clock out and notice that some of the time sheets have been written on in red ink. Hours worked had been documented in the bank holiday column, but had been scribbled out and put under the weekend column instead.

Bank holidays paid time and a half, but it was often difficult to decipher exactly what constituted a bank holiday in the eyes of the company. Boxing day would be paid at a normal working rate, or weekend rate if it fell on a weekend. The days after a public holiday such as Christmas or New Year, despite being classified as holiday in lieu, or an official bank holiday, were still not paid at the bank holiday rate to staff members. The only day that paid double time was Christmas day.

The management were often very evasive when asked about bank holidays, and the staff used to get angry, as many would think they were working for bank holiday rates, but find out at the end of the month that they had actually been working for either standard hourly rate or just weekend rate, despite some of the days being official bank holidays.

I walk out to my car, which has completely frozen up again with ice. I get out my ice scraper once again and start chiselling away at the windscreen. I look up at the pitch black sky, the stars twinkling away, a full moon radiating its brightness across the car park, and I wonder where my nursing will eventually take me, and the adventures and people I will come across. I was one day into my new career, and had many more days to go. I remembered back to my university days, everything I had learnt, everything I had been shown.

Could we really make a difference, and initiate change for the better, making people's lives better, improving their quality of life, or would it all be a constant battle of wills with policies and procedures, the constant battle of differing mind sets?

There was the constant reminder of the education/practice gap, being told that it was a very different world to being at university and this was the real world.

Would we make a difference?

Could I make a difference?

Epilogue

Within the past few months there had been a lot of changes at the home. Jennifer eventually had to step down from being acting manager, to take over control of the new day centre. The previous manager came back to her role, after a considerable amount of time off, owing to ill health. Once back, she started to kick the home back into gear, and rule with an iron fist. This had started to get up the carers' backs, and they were not happy with the way in which the new manager operated, despite her having almost thirty years experience as a general nurse. As the months went on, the bickering and backstabbing become more frequent. Some of the carers had started to put in complaints against the manager. They were not happy in how they were being spoken to. The owner jumped at the chance to offer any carer a chance to put in a formal grievance over this.

The grievances built up, and one rainy day in May, the manager made a quick tour of each of the units, in casual dress, with a small tear in her eye, and announced that she was leaving for good. It was a shock to some, but not to others. She hadn't got a job to go to, she was just taking time out to re-evaluate her life and decide where she wanted to go next. A lot of the staff were not surprised; they had an inkling she was on her way out, and the rumour mill had already started to spread the stories, that she was forced out of the company, despite building the home up over the past six years.

Jennifer was back, to ease into the space, immediately becoming the new manager of the home. Carers would already start to see a change in her mood and see a more hardened version of her former self.

Jenny and Emma were both off to pastures new. They had asked Paul privately for references, as they trusted him, and didn't want management to get wind of them going. They didn't like the way things were being run anyway, and preferred to leave quietly, without a fuss. Sharon and Katie stayed on with the company. Sharon continued to insidiously control the other carers and nurses as best she could, and continued to work to her own set of rules.

Once Jennifer found out about Jenny and Emma leaving, she immediately asked Paul why they hadn't got an official reference from her. She was furious that they hadn't come to her for a reference, and she argued with Paul that they needed official references from senior management, as this was a part of proper CQC regulations. Paul just nodded, and agreed not to write any more references for any staff members from that day onwards. Jenny and Emma confirmed that they could get a reference as long as it was from *any* professional *or* management. They were perfectly within their rights to have Paul write one for them. Paul got the impression that Jennifer just didn't like the way in which they went about leaving, not notifying her of their plans.

Jennifer asked numerous carers back, off other units, to come and work on Franklyn unit, but they refused on pure principle. These carers had been mucked about enough, and moved without their say so a number of months previously. The carers were starting to make a stand.

The latest rumour going around the smoking shelter was that the manager of Franklyn unit, Jodie, was going to run the day centre, leaving a space free for a member of staff to run Franklyn unit. Rumour had it that Jodie was only on fifty pence more an hour, as the clinical lead nurse in charge of the whole of Franklyn unit. Not a great deal of reward, for such a massive responsibility.

Paul had been looking for his own exit strategy. And one day, he found it. Paul eventually had enough of working as a nurse on the unit; he had become increasingly frustrated and anxious about the role. He walked onto the unit one morning, and started to shake and sweat. He couldn't do it any more. He felt ill every time he thought about working on the unit, especially if he was going to be the only nurse. He had enough of being pushed into every direction possible, hounded by the carers and the management. He was fed up with the paperwork and general bureaucracy. That morning he finally broke. He went straight to Jennifer and said that he just couldn't do the job any more. Jennifer asked him if he felt safe to work. He didn't. Jennifer immediately sent him home that day, and Paul took himself straight to the doctors.

Paul had two weeks off for depression, and took some time out to gather his thoughts about what he really wanted to do. When he returned back to the unit he had decided on his course of action. He was going to return, but as a carer. Jennifer immediately supported him in his wishes, and Paul began work again on Franklyn unit, on a carer's wage, doing three twelve hour shifts a week. He had much less responsibility, but that is what he wanted, and more importantly, no nursing paperwork to fill in. He immediately felt like a great weight had been lifted. He was doing more hours, but had less responsibility. He would still be there for any of the nurses to ask him advice, but as far as he was concerned, he would never work on Franklyn unit again as a qualified nurse.

I was looking for my own way out too; after over a year of being put upon and stressed out most days, I had really come to the end of my patience. It was time for a change. I had started to wake in the middle of the night in a cold sweat, dreaming about the place on numerous occasions, from being in that high stressed environment. Eventually no one seemed to value you any more as an individual. You were just a number to them, and as long as you played ball, you could be moulded and styled to however they wanted you to be, and pushed to your limit.

I had even asked to join the day care centre, but I was told that it would be a massive waste of my nursing skills, and that if I were to work there, then I would not be paid as a nurse, and would only be on a carer's wage. I had received my answer. They were not willing to accommodate me. The day centre was not doing as well as they would have liked. There were only three main members of staff who worked there, and the details of any residents using the facility were kept strictly under wraps. You could do great things there, I was sure. Getting relatives involved too, in support groups, and student nurses. Students were desperate to gain placement areas in the local hospice, even if it was just to do the gardening, but they were being turned away. If time is one of the crucial elements that is lacking in healthcare, then we should be embracing the skills and help from anyone who wishes to get involved.

To date there were no students working in the day centre. They had started to get student nurses on our unit, but as yet, not many had passed through the units. It was a slow roll out, but it had started to happen. We have to look to our other resources and all work together in creating a unified front, helping and caring for our residents in the best way we can.

Relatives are often a very useful resource, and one that we do not always appreciate. Many relatives would come onto Franklyn unit at mealtimes, and help feed their husband or wife. Some carers would see them as a hindrance, and see them as getting in the way. But they could be a huge help to the effective running of the unit, and also to the well being of others. Many a relative would also engage with the other residents, and talk to them, whilst also being with their significant others. Even such a small amount of input could help hugely during the course of a twelve hour shift.

If time is the main factor in why we cannot be with our residents as much as we would like, then we should be embracing everyone we can who can afford even a few moments of their time to engage and help out. People like Deirdre, who would spend her time doing the laundry every single day, and washing medicine pots, would carry on like this, each and every day, without a complaint in the world, whilst her husband slowly deteriorated in his bed. It is here that we need to be looking a little more intrinsically outside of 'the box', working together in harmony and doing the best we can, with what resources we do have. It is often easy to criticise things we do not have, whilst not appreciating things we do have, and can do.

I had also requested training in management numerous times, requesting to do an NVQ 4 in management. Interestingly when I dug out my original person specification for the job it specifically stated 'must be willing to work towards an NVQ 4 in management'. I had been brushed off and they were not willing to pay to train me in management. It made sense, I guess. All the managers were in post, and not likely to be moving on any time soon. There was nowhere else to go in the company.

I had tried to think of numerous options, but they were all rejected. Whilst money wasn't a deciding factor on where you wished to work, the home was strictly carrying on, not offering anyone a pay rise in over two years. I had begun to join various nursing agencies, but they had all come back with the same answers: more nursing homes, and not much else. It was clear where the demand was, and where it would continue to be. My phone would often ring two to three times a day with job offers at these homes.

I had also heard through various sources that the RGN's were respected more than the RMN's and that they were paid a higher hourly rate as they were considered to have more all round knowledge in more physical health areas. The RMN's were there as a legal requirement, but many thought that it was the RGN's who were really running things. My manager had continued to deny this alleged discrepancy in pay. It was also a known fact that the home manager had also had a recent pay rise for her dedication to her new role, whilst all other staff members in the home remained on the same hourly rate.

I had tried my best, and given my all, but sometimes you just have to cut your losses and look at your own well being, and mental health, and look for pastures new. I know there is something out there that would better suit my skills and experience, and I appreciate the time I was able to spend with my residents, and hope that I made a small difference in their lives. I had tried, and that was all I could do. It was now time to close the book on nursing homes, and start a new chapter.

Burn out

After almost two years working in the nursing home, it had finally zapped me of all my energy and will. I found it a struggle to get up of a morning, let alone walk through those doors once more and face the stress of the unit as a whole. I had tried appraisals and supervision with my manager, but they hadn't listened.

They had said I was continuing to do a good job and that they were shocked by some of the issues I had raised.

There was no room for promotion as everyone was in place. The money was never going to increase. Where was the motivation to improve your skills and development if you knew you were never going to go up any form of pay scale.

I had begun to suffer some anxieties and stress on a daily basis. I used to get horrific night terrors. Every single night I would dream of the place; residents would infiltrate my dreams, and I would see them walking towards me holding out their withered hands, asking for my help. Each morning I would have a terrible heavy feeling weighing down on my mind, causing my stomach to creak. The drive to the home became more and more difficult, trying to imagine what was in store for me.

The start of the pressures had begun when they had started to run the unit with only one nurse for the whole of the shift, and mainly only four staff members including me. I simply couldn't get off the unit for any considerable amount of time without either being called back for an emergency, or worrying throughout my break at the thought of something going wrong.

I would frequently work from 8 a.m. till around 2:30 – 3 p.m. without ever having a single break. The carers always got their break, and would always stress and make sure that they always had one. They never usually noticed about the nurse. I was quite sure that some of them expected the nurse not to be entitled to one as we were getting paid more than them.

I used to worry about residents getting sicker, relatives

becoming more demanding, and every time one came up to me to ask about their relative I would instantly panic, and feel a wave of stress instantly hit me. I was close to burn out. I could feel it building, day upon day. Mental health really hadn't seemed this linear and task orientated when I was a student.

Nurses were being used as pawns. You were there to administer medication that you may not agree with, to support the carers as much as you could, and to spend little time with the people that mattered, the residents. I would fight my cause, and try to spend as much time as possible with them, even if that meant a few stolen minutes during the medication round in the morning. I realised my time was done in this area. I had hoped I had made a small difference to the lives of the residents, but the pressures upon me from all areas had become too much. I myself had become borderline depressed, and saw my three years of training being used for nothing more than a number on a nursing home's employee list.

I saw my future as no more than twenty years stuck in a home, never being able to develop my skills or introduce change, becoming more and more ill with stress, and watching the owners getting richer and richer, whilst my wages never moved.

I would always miss my residents, and there had been some truly genuine good times there, but as all the good carers slowly left one by one, and more stresses were put upon you as a nurse, including more and more paperwork that you could never hope to complete, it had become a daily grind, and that wasn't fair on anyone, especially the residents. This was a job where your heart had to be in it, and mine just wasn't. So I did the right thing.

I eventually had to go off work sick with stress. I went to the doctor and he agreed that I should be signed off for a minimum of two weeks. The home had broken me, just like it had Paul. Only I was right at the start of my career. I am not someone who caves into pressure and the stresses of a job easily, but even I had my breaking point. I couldn't bear the sense of dread before each shift, wondering who would be off sick, what problems would arise throughout the day. During my time off my head became a lot clearer. I had started to feel a lot better, and I realised that if I was to be true to myself and my own well being then I had to leave.

This was the first time I had ever had to go to a doctor's for anything like this. Sure, I had jobs in the past that I didn't like, but they were bearable. This was something else, something I had never encountered before, and it scared me, the powerful and detrimental impact it was having on my own mental health.

I had tried to find other jobs, in other areas, but it was a real uphill struggle. With final desperation I decided to do a bit of temping work at another nursing home not too far from me, just to get some additional experience. Despite it being the same area, I figured I had to try something, just to get out of where I was. They eventually offered me a twenty four hour contract which I accepted. The next stage was to see if I could still work a twelve hour shift at my current home, giving me experience in two different areas. Many of the carers often had their shifts moved around and hours raised or lowered, so I didn't see any potential problems. I booked an appointment to go and see Jennifer and discuss it, bright and early after a previous night shift (running two units, and being responsible for forty residents).

I walked into the office. Jennifer was busy at her

computer, already amending what appeared to be next month's rota. A pile of paperwork was strewn lazily all over the desk.

'Jack, do come in.'

Before I could sit down properly, she immediately quizzed me.

'So where are you working?'

I tell her the name of the new home.

'Right, the problem I have is, you have a full time contract, and that's to fulfil full time hours. If I'm honest twelve hours is just not going to be useful to me or the company. And the day you have picked means that is the doctors' round, and you simply won't have the knowledge or have been on the unit enough in order to lead it.'

'Okay, well what about another day? Or maybe even an eighteen hour contract?'

'It still won't be enough. I'm going to be very honest with you; I'm not trying to box you in a corner here, even though it may seem like it, but you are going to have to make a decision. I can't have a nurse working in two places, and potentially doing more hours, and being tired.'

'I wouldn't be, it's only a twenty four hour contract that I have been promised.'

'Well I don't know that!'

'So there is no movement at all then?'

'No, and I sense you are going to move, as you're probably fed up, so if you do, I will need it in writing to terminate your contract.'

'Well, I haven't actually decided yet, I'm just being honest with you, and considering my options.'

'I understand, and that's why I'm being equally honest back to you.'

'And the other thing, if I'm being honest, is money. There hasn't been a pay rise in over two years, are you the right person to speak to about that? Is there room for any negotiation over that?'

'Listen Jack, with regards to your recent appraisal, it is clear that you are struggling a little with responsibility and confidence. We don't pay people extra unless they are taking on more responsibility, there is no more money in the pot. I know the home you are working at pays more, but then they are a much bigger company, and a pay rise is not something I will be able to offer.'

'Right, so it seems pretty clear then.'

'All I will say to you is, you have to do what you think is right for you, it's your decision. This home won't collapse without you. I will just need to know what you are doing, so I can recruit again.'

She rolls her eyes at the thought of recruitment.

'I've spoken to the owner, and I'm afraid it's final, it's stay with us, or move on, your decision. If you do move on now though, it will have particular implications for the courses that we have paid for you to do, and you would have to pay us back.'

I had opted to commence two dementia courses with my local university; no such thing as a free lunch. I had to sign a disclaimer to say I would pay back the fees if I left the company within eighteen months.

'No, I understand. I have a lot to think about.'

'Right, now if you will excuse me, I'm busy preparing a sheet for the Thai cleaners, as they were fighting outside my door yesterday, so I'm writing some clear instructions which I am going to translate online about how I expect them to behave around here!'

I left the office. The meeting hadn't exactly gone to plan. I was hoping I would feel a valued member of the team, and that they would want me to stay, and try to accommodate that. Jennifer had basically told me I was easily expendable, and replaceable, hinting that I couldn't handle the stresses and responsibility of the job, despite these main stresses coming directly from the company short staffing (minimal numbers) the unit, and lacking support for its nurses, refusing me to work at the day centre, and turning down my requests to be trained up on the NVQ management scheme.

The only real training I had done was upon my request, and I had to sign a waiver for that. It was a shame; even one of the home's newsletters had stated that they are 'always keen to hear from any members of staff who want to try new opportunities if they arise', and they will 'do our very best to accommodate changes within the home if at all possible'. This didn't appear possible in my case.

I handed in my notice, and left, finally closing the book on my nursing home experiences. I never looked back. Jennifer reaffirmed what I already knew; she told me directly that I wasn't going to go anywhere in this company as it was a small company. It wasn't always as easy as you thought to leave. I had managed to see my reference, written by Jennifer. It had stated that I sometimes lacked confidence in running a unit, but she had no problems with me running one.

I fared better than a previous colleague, who had been with the company six months. She stated on his official reference 'lacks motivation and enthusiasm, unsure I would employ him again'. It seemed they really didn't like people to leave, especially to another similar establishment. A rather subjective opinion on someone that could be deemed in certain situations as a defamation of character.

In the past Jennifer had rung ahead to the ex employees' new workplace to fill the new employers in on her ex staffs' behaviour. The new employers would often ignore her, but it just showed you how far they were willing to go to potentially tarnish a good reputation.

I still miss my residents. When I left I realised that I was actually appreciated by a lot of the relatives too. I received many gifts from them, and they had said very kind words in their thank you cards, one thanking me for all the time I gave their dad, another for all the kindness and care I had shown towards them. Despite all the challenges of the unit, I had managed to make a small difference, in at least some people's eyes.

Why My Care Plans were never up to date

In the end, the pressure had got so bad that I felt I had to justify myself to any potential managers, auditors, or inspectors as to why a lot of my key jobs were not getting done. This is what I wrote, in case I ever needed a true justification of why my nursing duties were falling behind;

- Franklyn unit is frequently staffed to minimum staffing levels, as per the RCN minimum staff recommendations of 1 member of staff to 5 residents, allowing a minimum of 4 members of staff (including the nurse) at any one time.

- The unit is frequently run on 4 members of staff. RCN policy position on evidence based nurse staffing levels (2010) states: 'Services and the staff required to provide them must be shaped on the basis of patient need.' I feel they are more based on the minimum recommendations and financial costing.

- As a nurse I am expected to help out 'on the floor' as much as possible, including helping with morning drinks, putting people to bed, and helping feed. I have been told this numerous times by my immediate line manager and lead dementia manager.

- There is consistent pressure from the carers to help out on a daily basis, no matter what other nursing duties may arise during the day.

- I am paid as a RMN. At times it feels I am doing more of a carer's job, and not being able to fulfil all my RMN duties due to these pressures.

- When the unit is run on 4 staff, quality of care is considerably compromised, carers 'rush' and become more 'task based', and at times will put residents to bed early to appease their own time keeping and running of the unit.

- No activities are done in the afternoon time; residents do not get enough quality time and are not offered enough opportunities for stimulating activities or therapies. There is only one activities co-ordinator who rarely visits the unit.

- There are a lot of residents who frequently wander up and down the unit on a daily basis. Without enough staff members, these residents cannot be afforded the time to distract them or take them out off the unit in order to achieve additional stimulation.

- Without stimulation and one on one time with residents, some residents get increasingly anxious and agitated. These residents often have their medication increased or put on new medication and anti-psychotics. The Banerjee report (2009) states ' Where intervention is needed, psychological approaches such as structured social interaction should be used in the first instance'. There is not enough time afforded to utilise such psychological approaches due to the pressures of the unit.

A resident who was frequently wandering and agitated and grabbing hold of female residents has been put on Benperidol, a powerful anti-psychotic and sexual inappropriateness drug. No thought was given to structured social interaction or a non medical intervention prior to this decision.

- As a nurse I feel guilty for trying to spend just 5-10 minutes with any of my residents, as there is a frequent pressure to 'get on with things' and help out as much as possible. Barker (2001) lists many other reasons for not spending time with residents in The Tidal Model: 'Too busy - keeping the ward safe, too busy - 'fire fighting' and crisis management, too busy on the phone in the office.'

- I have had complaints in the past for not answering the phone enough. The phone goes frequently throughout the day and often during key times, such as medication rounds and mealtimes. The phone on the unit can ring on average around 30-40 times a day. Being the only nurse in charge means I have to deal with most of these phone calls.

- The unit has now moved towards just one nurse being in charge, meaning all responsibility is down to me. This means I have to speak to all relatives who may ring or visit, be involved in ward rounds, and deal with any other medical emergencies. I am still counted in the numbers as part of the minimum staff recommendations of 4, and I am still expected to help out with the carers on the floor.

- My stress levels have considerably risen as a result. The RCN define stress as 'the adverse reaction people have to excessive pressure or other types of demand placed on them'. I have expressed my concerns numerous times about being the only nurse in charge and told it 'will be good experience'.

- I am responsible for six residents' care plans and updating.

- The monthly rota now indicates a day each month for time off the floor to do my care plans. This has not happened for over four months due to the unit being staffed at minimum levels, and high sick rates, meaning I have had to stay on the unit to run it.

- When other professionals need to see my care plans for CHC funding assessments and dementia reviews, it looks bad on me as a professional and not the home.

- It is all nurses on the unit who are frequently behind with their care plans and updating, including my manager.

- When some of my care plans are written, at times they have been destroyed, despite them being legal documentation, and rewritten by the lead dementia manager. This has made me feel undermined in my role. In this case a resident who could eat a normal diet was put onto pureed foods as a result, despite her being able to maintain a healthy and nutritious diet with normal foods. The carers all agreed that they couldn't understand why my care plan had been destroyed rather than updated. The resident has since continued to enjoy a balanced and nutritious normal diet.

- When the lead dementia manager does an audit and finds the paperwork is out of date we are told to not help out on the floor as much and concentrate on our paperwork to get it all up to date to look good for an audit. The demands are still there, and it is frequently very difficult to grab time away to write them.

- I frequently miss my breaks due to the constraints and demands of the unit. This puts more pressure and stress on me as a nurse to keep the unit running smoothly, whilst slowly affecting my own mental health and wellbeing.

These are why my care plans are not up to date

Did you change your view of what mental health is like? Do the images that you conjured up in your mind bear any resemblance to what was described? I hope that at least this has given you a true understanding of what it is like to work in these typical conditions, and how dementia is on a daily basis. The media can report on issues and the Government can produce numerous reports, but what really matters is our residents, and how we can help them. What is working, and what isn't.

It isn't simple, and I don't have all the answers, no one does, but I can at least show you a small glimpse into my world, and show you what it is like, and the barriers that sometimes stand in our way. Without forward thinking and assertiveness, we will never be able to challenge the system, and fight for improvement. It won't be easy, but we have to start somewhere.

I can only spread my message through the written word and in my practice. I hope that you will join me on my journey to improvement. And just remember, one day it might be someone you know who has dementia, a friend or family member.

One day it could be you or I. How would you like to be treated? How would you like to be cared for? What decisions would you like to be made about your medication? These are all important questions, and we all have to work together if we are going to challenge and improve health care, one step at a time.

References

Adams, T., (2005), Communication and interaction within dementia care triads: Developing a theory for relationship centred care, <u>Dementia</u>, Vol 4, (2), pp185-205

Andrews, J., (2010), Imaginative Care, <u>Nursing Standard</u>, (24),(37) p61, RCN Publishing Company Ltd, Middlesex

Alzheimer's Society, (2011), Drug treatments for Alzheimer's disease, available from: http://alzheimers.org.uk/site/scripts/documents_info.php?documentID=147

British Heart Foundation, (2011), <u>What is Blood Pressure?</u>, available from:

http://www.bhf.org.uk/heart-health/conditions/high-blood-pressure.aspx

Banerjee, S., (2009), <u>The use of antipsychotic medication for people with dementia: Time for action</u>, Department of Health, London

Barker P. (2001). "The Tidal Model: developing an empowering, person-centred approach to recovery within psychiatric and mental health nursing." *Journal of Psychiatric and Mental Health Nursing* **8**: 233-240.

BBC News, (2012), Depression drugs 'causing falls', {Online},Available at: http://www.bbc.co.uk/news/health-16618160

Caring Matters, (2005), Defining Relationship – Centred Care,

Available: http://www.caringmatters.com/html/DefiningRCC.htm

Cummings, J., Emre, M., Aarsland, D., Tekin, S., Dronamraju, N., Lane, R., (2010), Effects of rivastigmine in Alzheimer's disease patients with and without hallucinations, <u>Journal of Alzheimers Disease</u>, 20, (1), pp 301-311

Directgov, (2011), <u>What is lasting power of attorney?</u>, available from:

http://www.direct.gov.uk/en/Governmentcitizensandrights/Mentalcapacityandthelaw/Mentalcapacityandplanningahead/DG_185921

Gold Standards Framework Centre, (2005), <u>Prognostic Indicator Guidance Paper</u>, Gold Standards Framework, London.

Harrow Council, (2011), Safeguarding Adults Services: Institutional Abuse, Available from:

http://www.harrow.gov.uk/info/731/protectionof vulnerable adults/973/safeguarding adults services/1

Ministry of Health and Long Term Care, (2009), Committee to Evaluate Drugs (CED): Rivastigmine Patch,: Recommendations and Reasons, available from: http://www.health.gov.on.ca/english/providers/program/drugs/ced/pdf/exelon_patch.pdf

National Institute for Health and Clinical Excellence, (2010), Alzheimer's disease – donepezil, galantamine, rivastigmine and memantine (review): appraisal consultation document, Available from: http://www.nice.org.uk/guidance/index.jsp?action=article&o=51047

NHS Your Choice Magazine, (2011), How To Avoid a Facebook Folly, Autumn Edition, p113, Combined Media Ltd, Cheshire,
available from: http://www.nhsmagazine.net/sth/

NHS Choices, (2011), What is NHS Continuing Healthcare? available from:

http://www.nhs.uk/chq/Pages/2392.aspx?CategoryID=68&SubCategoryID=681

Nursing and Midwifery Council, (2008), <u>The Code: Standards for conduct, performance and ethics for nurses and midwives</u>, London: NMC

Nursing and Midwifery Council, (2009), <u>Guidance for the care of older people</u>, London, NMC

<u>Nursing Times</u>, (2011), Nurses fear for patient safety, (107), (37), p2, Emap, London.

<u>Nursing Times</u>, (2011), Social networking: avoiding the pitfalls, (107), (37), P15, Emap, London

Torjesen, I., Waters, A., (2010), Men on a mission, <u>Nursing Standard</u>, (24), (37), pp20-22, RCN Publishing Company Ltd, Middlesex

Parliamentary and Health Service Ombudsman, (2011), <u>Care and compassion ? Report of the Health Service Ombudsman on ten investigations into NHS care of older people</u>, The Stationary Office, London

Royal College of Nursing, (2010), <u>Guidance on safe nurse staffing levels in the UK</u>, Policy Unit, London

Royal College of Nursing, (2010), <u>RCN policy position: evidence-based nurse staffing levels</u>, Royal College of Nursing, London

Schneider, L.S, Tariot, P.N, Dagerman, K.S, Davis, S.M, Hsiao, J.K, Ismail, M.S, Lebowitz, B.D, Lyketsoos, C.G, Ryan, J.M, Stroup, T.S, Sultzer, D.L, Weintraub, D., Lieberman, J.A, Catie, A.D Study Group, (2006) Effectiveness of atypical antipsychotic drugs in patients with Alzheimer's disease, New England Journal of Medicine, Oct 12: 355 (15); pp1525-38

Waugh, A. & Grant, A. (2004) Ross and Wilson Anatomy and Physiology in Health and Illness: 9th edition. Edinburgh, Elsevier.

World Health Organisation, (1993), The ICD-10 Classification of Mental and Behavioural Disorders: Diagnostic criteria for research, World Health Organization, Geneva

Don't Mention Dementia